DELIVERING HEALTH CARE TO HOMELESS PERSONS

THE DIAGNOSIS AND MANAGEMENT OF MEDICAL AND MENTAL HEALTH CONDITIONS

David Wood, MD, MPH, is currently a pediatrician on faculty at the University of California at Los Angeles (UCLA) and Cedars Sinai Medical Center in Los Angeles, and Medical Director of the Los Angeles Homeless Health Care Project. He has been delivering health services to homeless families for more than 5 years.

Delivering Health Care to Homeless Persons

The Diagnosis and Management of Medical and Mental Health Conditions

David Wood, MD, MPH
Editor

SPRINGER PUBLISHING
New York

Springer Publishing Company, Inc.
536 Broadway
New York, NY 10012

92 93 94 95 96 / 5 4 3 2 1

Delivering health care to homeless persons : The diagnosis and
    management of medical and mental health conditions / David
    Wood, editor.
        p.   cm.
    "This publication was developed under the auspices of the Los
Angeles Homeless Health Care Project"—Acknowledgments.
    Includes bibliographical references and index.
    ISBN 0-8261-7780-8
    1. Homeless persons—Medical care—United States. 2. Homeless
persons—Mental health services—United States. I. Wood, David,
1955–   . II. Los Angeles Homeless Health Care Project.
    [DNLM: 1. Delivery of Health Care—United States. 2. Homeless
Persons. 3. Primary Health Care. W 84.6 D355]
    RA564.9.H63D45   1992
    362.1'0425—dc20
    DNLM/DLC
    for Library of Congress   91-5074
                                                                  CIP

Printed in the United States of America

Contents

Acknowledgments

This publication was developed under the auspices of the Los Angeles Homeless Health Care Project. We wish to acknowledge the support of the Board of Directors, and the contributions of the staff, Al Shen, Marjorie Sa'adah, and, especially, Pamela Thompson, whose assistance in typing, organizing, and coordinating this manuscript have been invaluable to its successful completion.

We also wish to acknowledge the National Association of Community Health Centers, and the Bureau of Health Care Delivery and Assistance, particularly Freda Mitchum and Joan Holloway, for their support of this project.

Lastly, we would like to acknowledge the diligent work and many long hours of attention given to the project by Gerri Dallek, MPH. Her thoughtful input made many significant contributions to the final manuscript.

Contributors

Robin K. Avery, MD, is a Fellow in the Division of Infectious Diseases, Department of Medicine, and Instructor at Harvard Medical School.

Mark Casanova is a Family Therapist and Family Case Manager for the Los Angeles Homeless Health Care Project (LAHHCP).

Michael R. Cousineau, DrPH, is the Director of the LAHHCP, which oversees outreach, training, and case management programs among the homeless.

Robert Erlenbusch is a Director for the West Hollywood Homeless Health Program.

Tom Farnham, MD, is the Medical Director of the homeless outreach project at the Community Health Foundation of East Los Angeles.

Susan Fleischman, MD, is an Assistant Clinical Professor at UCLA, Department of Medicine, and Director of Medical Services at the Venice Family Clinic. At the clinic she has been involved in the care of homeless clients as well as teaching residence about medical care for homeless persons.

Jennifer Garshman, MD, is Assistant Professor of Pediatrics and Psychiatry, University of Massachusetts Medical Center. She worked with homeless and high-risk adolescents during her fellowship at the Childrens Hospital of Los Angeles and the University of Southern California.

Lillian Gelberg, MD, MSPH, is Assistant Professor in the Department of Family Medicine at UCLA. She has conducted several surveys of homeless populations, and has published several articles on the physical and mental health of homeless persons.

Joanne Jubelier is a licensed psychologist and has served as a consultant to the Venice Family Clinics' Homeless Health Care Project since 1985, providing counseling and psychosocial services at shelters and clinics. She is also a psychotherapist in private practice.

Paul Koegel, PhD, is a Research Anthropologist at the Rand Corporation. He has been involved in research on homelessness and mental illness since 1984, first conducting a psychiatric epidemiological survey of inner-city homeless adults in Los Angeles and more recently carrying out an ethnographical examination of the ongoing lives of homeless mentally ill adults.

James R. Lockyer, MD, is a Clinical Instructor on the faculty of University of Southern California School of Medicine in the Department of Internal Medicine. He is Medical Director of the Weingart Center Clinic, which serves the homeless population of the Los Angeles Skid Row area.

Richard G. MacKenzie, MD, is Director of Adolescent Medicine, Childrens Hospital of Los Angeles, and Associate Professor of Pediatrics and Medicine, University of Southern California School of Medicine, and has worked with homeless and high-risk adolescents through clinics and outreach programs at the Childrens Hospital of Los Angeles.

Elizabeth McNally, RN, FNP, is a Family Nurse Practitioner at the Stout Street Clinic in Denver, Colorado. She has developed a unique practice approach with homeless women that provides prenatal care and delivery services.

James J. O'Connell, MD, is Director of the Boston Health Care for the Homeless Program. He is an instructor in Medicine at Harvard Medical School and is a member of the General Medicine Unit of Massachusetts General Hospital.

Claire B. Panosian, MD, DTM&H, is an assistant Clinical Professor of Medicine, Division of Infectious Diseases, Department of Medicine, UCLA School of Medicine.

Charlene G. Sanders, MD, is Attending Physician in the Divisions of Adolescent Medicine and Emergency Medicine, Childrens Hospital of Los Angeles, and Clinical Professor of Pediatrics, University of Southern California of Medicine, and has worked with homeless and high-risk adolescents through clinics and outreach programs at the Childrens Hospital of Los Angeles.

Daniel Sherman, PhD, is a clinical psychologist at Skid Row Mental Health Center which serves homeless mentally ill adults in skid row, Los Angeles.

Mary H. Smith, FNP-C, MSN, a Family Nurse Practitioner at the Venice Family Clinic, supervises the clinic's homeless outreach program. She has been working on homeless health care programs for 5 years.

Richard Usatine, MD, is an Assistant Professor in the Department of Family Medicine at UCLA. He served for 4 years as a clinician at the Venice Family Clinic and helped direct its homeless medical program.

Linda Weinreb, MD, is an Assistant Professor, Department of Family and Community Medicine, University of Massachusetts Medical School, and Medical Director at the Better Homes Foundation. Dr. Weinreb has directed neighborhood-based clinic programs for homeless persons in San Francisco, California, and Worcester, Massachusetts. She has provided clinical care to homeless adults and families for the past 8 years.

Julie Wood RN, PHN, is a Public Health Nurse for the Los Angeles County Public Health Department. She works at the largest family shelter in Los Angeles and is active in providing prenatal care to pregnant homeless women.

Gary L. Yates, MA, MFCC, is Associate Director, Division of Adolescent Medicine, Childrens Hospital of Los Angeles.

Introduction

The American health care system in the United States is a paradox of excess and deprivation. Americans spend more on health care per capital than any other nation, and many people benefit from advanced technologies and elaborate therapeutic interventions. Yet, 37 million Americans have no health insurance, and many of these people are denied the most basic of health services. The American health care system is a patchwork quilt of independent medical providers, hospitals, clinics, long-term care agencies, managed care systems, third-party payers, and consumers. The loosely defined and poorly coordinated relationships between health institutions, professionals, and health care workers have caused many to refer to "our nonsystem of care" in the United States that empahsizes cure over prevention, and technology over concern for social causes of injury and disease; indeed, America has no equal in keeping a low-birthweight baby alive but has been unable to extend the benefits of prenatal care to all pregnant women. Highly technical surgical procedures and medicines have been developed for rare disorders, whereas easily cured diseases such as syphilis and gonorhea remain unchecked.

The American medical system is anything but user friendly for most Americans. Low-income patients, in particular, must make their way through a complicated maze of institutional barriers to care. Patients encounter complex insurance forms and regulations; large, bureaucratic, and impersonal medical centers; and few of the supportive services they need to enhance recovery. All of these barriers make access to care for the nation's poor, difficult, if not impossible.

No group has more difficulty obtaining care than the homeless. As many as 3 million men, women, and children are homeless today in America. The homeless represent a cross section of impoverished people for whom housing has become a critical issue. Millions of Americans spend well over 50% of their income on rent; for these families and individuals, a crisis, such as a health problem, loss of a job, or loss of welfare assistance, will push them into the streets and into the cycle of homelessness. The health problems of homeless people are well documented. Nevertheless, extreme poverty, lack of insurance (including Medicaid), mental illness, and alcohol and other drug abuse are but a few of the reasons homeless people are undesirable to most health care providers. The homeless are America's pariahs.

This book is about providing health care to the homeless of America. It describes the innovative approaches developed to serve this population, and ways to manage the particular medical conditions and problems encountered in homeless adults and children. Health care for the homeless demands a new way of looking at the delivery of medical care. By necessity, this system of care must be patient centered and not provider centered. It requires reaching out to places where the homeless live and congregate, as well as providing case management for the diverse and unique medical, social, and psychological needs of the population. Finally, as so many of the authors of this book point out, caring for the homeless requires a special compassion and patience.

The outreach-oriented health services to the homeless persons described in this book were pioneered nationally in 1985 under a 19-city demonstration project sponsored by the Robert Wood Johnson Foundation, the PEW Charitable Trusts, and the U.S. Conference of Mayors. The goal of the national demonstration project was to establish effective models of delivery of primary health care to the homeless. The model was later expanded to include a greater empahsis on mental health and substance abuse services.

In 1987 the federal Stewart B. McKinney Act established a new Section 340 of the Public Health Service Act and expanded the 19-city demonstration to 109 projects. This funding has enabled close to 100 community and migrant health centers, and 60 health departments, hospitals, and other nonprofit health care organizations to establish the outreach and case management capabilities needed to provide off-site delivery of health services to homeless people. Services are provided in soup kitchens, emergency shelters, welfare hotels, and on the streets, while at the same time working to integrate these patients into ongoing systems of care in their communities. During the first year of operation, McKinney programs served 232,000 homeless patients through 783,000 patient encounters.

To assist with implementation of the McKinney-funded Health Care for the Homeless programs, the U.S. Bureau of Health Care Delivery and Assistance provided funding to the Washington, D.C.-based National Association of Community Health Center (NACHC) to conduct a national training and capacity-building program for homeless health care providers. As part of this training effort, NACHC provided funding support for the development of this book.

This book is directed toward (a) nurses, midlevel practitioners, physicians, and other health personnel who see the homeless on a regular basis and want some experienced guidance on diagnosis and management of health problems; and (b) practitioners who see homeless persons on an irregular or occasional basis to help them understand the special medical, social, and psychological problems found among homeless persons and enable them to manage their medical care more effectively.

This book is not a medical textbook. Much of the specifics of the diagnosis, treatment, and management of diseases discussed in the book are assumed to be within the clinical knowledge of the reader. Rather, this book seeks to describe the medical and social considerations important in the treatment of homeless persons. The environment of homelessness affects the clinician-patient relationship in such a way that medicine must be practiced in a different way. Many accepted standards of practiced medicine are ineffective in the setting of homelessness. In this book the authors, all of whom have worked in homeless health care settings, describe how traditional medical care should be modified. At times the clinician must depart from accepted standards of practice and creatively adapt medicine to the need of the patient.

This book does not advocate for an institutionalized system of care for the homeless of America, however. Clearly, such a system would remain at the bottom of a multitiered system of care for which there would be few advocates; none of the authors believes that delivering health care on the streets or in shelters is an optimal way of caring for seriously ill people. It contradicts many of our own commitments to promote the best quality of care for our patients. We recognize that the actual causes of the disorders addressed in this book are in large part social and environmental in nature. Therefore, resolving and preventing health problems among the homeless are ultimately policy questions mired in the underlying causes of homelessness itself: lack of affordable housing, a fragmented health care system that leaves out millions, and a disintegrating safety net for the poor.

This book has four parts: Part I—Overview, Part II—Medical Issues, Part III—Pediatric and Maternal Health Issues, and Part IV—Mental Health Issues.

The first part begins with an ethnography by Drs. Koegel and Gelbert that gives an insightful glimpse into the lives of three patients served by homeless health projects. Next, Dr. Gelberg summarizes the now extensive literature on the physical and mental health status and special risk factors of homeless persons. In Chapter 3, Dr. Cousineau, Casanova, and Erlenbush present an overview of case management for homeless persons as it is applied in the health service setting. In Chapter 4, Smith describes how a health center can design and implement comprehensive and triage clinics at locations beyond the health center where the homeless congregate. Finally, Dr. Weinreb details the importance of preventive health procedures among the homeless and how to incorporate them into ongoing medical care for homeless persons.

The second part of the book focuses on adult medical issues and begins with a discussion by Drs. Fleischman and Farnham of the commonest chronic diseases encountered among the homeless. Next, Dr. Lockyer describes the assessment and treatment considerations for alcohol and drug abuse in the homeless. In Chapter 8, Drs. Avery and O'Connell describe the medical evaluation and management of AIDS among homeless adults, and offer guidelines on screening and support services. Chapter 9 by Dr. Fleischman describes the common traumatic injuries sustained by homeless adults and how a clinic can coordinate the management of trauma care with local emergency rooms. Dr. Usatine then presents the common dermatologic problems diagnosed among the homeless, their presentation, and management. Chapter 11 by Dr. Lockyer is a description of the diagnostic and management subtleties of the very common problem of hypothermia among the homeless. Finally, Dr. Panosian presents the epidemiology and special treatment considerations pertinent to tuberculosis among the homeless.

The third part of the book has three chapters on maternal and child health issues among the homeless. In Chapter 13, McNally and Wood present the unique management considerations for homeless pregnant women. In Chapter 14, Dr. Wood then describes a profile of problems encountered in homeless children and presents a method for their clinical evaluation.

The last part of the book addresses the diagnosis and management of mental health problems of the homeless. Chapter 15 is a discussion by Drs. Garshman, Sanders, Yates, and MacKenzie of the diagnosis and management of health and mental problems common to homeless adolescents. Dr. Jubilier then describes the unique presentation of mental illness among homeless children and their parents, and gives guidelines for their management by a clinic-based mental health team. In the last chapter, Drs. Koegel and Sherman present the constraints inherent in the diagnosis and management of mental illness among adult homeless persons, and describe optimal diagnosis and management approaches.

A special acknowledgment should be made of the following practitioners in community health centers of other BHCDA (Bureau of Health Care Delivery and Assistance) programs whose reviews and comments helped make this book more relevant to the practicing clinician; Joann Lukomnik, MD, Irwin Redlener, MD, Ketty Gonzalez, MD, Marc Babitz, MD, Ken Schacter, MD, Roberta Holder Moseley, CNMW, Laurie Kunches, RN, NP, John Mozzule, MD, Ramon Torres, MD, Anita Vaughn, MD, Peter C. S. d'Aubermont, MD, and Patricia Salomon, MD.

Overview

Health of the Homeless: Definition of Problem

Lillian Gelberg

1

CHAPTER HIGHLIGHTS

- Empirical studies of the homeless are limited because of inherent problems in accurately sampling, defining, quantifying, and describing the homeless population.
- In comparison with the general population, the homeless have high rates of many categories of illness including hypertension, diabetes and its complications, skin problems, upper-respiratory illness, and communicable diseases.
- Depending on the population of homeless studied and the definition used, estimates of mental illness among the homeless population range from 16% to 91%.
- The homeless are less likely to obtain outpatient services, but more likely to be hospitalized for medical and psychiatric problems than the general population.
- The homeless encounter major obstacles in obtaining needed medical and psychiatric services including lack of money, long distance to care, disabling mental illness, inappropriate services, and the unwillingness of some providers to care for this population.

INTRODUCTION

Nationwide, at least 250,000 and as many as 3 million (Hombs & Snyder, 1982) people are estimated to be without a home. Given the large and growing numbers of homeless in the United States, health care providers, medical educators, and health services researchers are faced with the need to design and provide medical care to these individuals. To provide homeless persons with the most appropriate and effective health care, we must gain a greater awareness and understanding of the primary issues related to their physical and mental health. The purpose of this chapter is to describe what is currently known about the health of the homeless: their physical, dental, and mental health; risk factors for illness; use of health services; and barriers to obtaining health care. This information is based on a review of the literature on homelessness listed in MED-LINE through October 1988.

LIMITATIONS OF THE LITERATURE

Before describing what is known about the health of homeless persons, it is important to understand the limitations of the available literature. The empirical studies on the homeless are limited because of inherent problems in accurately defining, quantifying, and describing the homeless population. In coping with these difficulties, studies have used differing methodologies. They have differed on their definition of homelessness; sampling location (e.g., city, site type, clinical versus community setting, season, and prevailing weather); method of data collection (e.g., structured or unstructured interview, record review, or physical examination); and measurement of health (e.g., self-report, ratings, or objective data) (Baxter & Hopper, 1981; Levine, 1984).

Because there is no generally recognized definition of homelessness, studies have often focused on different subgroups of the homeless population. Many surveys of the homeless have sampled only the most accessible homeless (Farr, Koegel, & Burnam, 1987; Robertson, Ropers, & Boyer, 1985; Rossi, Wright, Fisher, et al., 1987)—those from emergency shelters or cheap hotels (single room occupancy hotels [SROs]). Researchers believe, however, that these individuals constitute only a small fraction of the homeless population in some parts of our country (e.g., fewer than 10% in Los Angeles County (Robertson, Ropers, & Boyer, 1984). Thus, the results of studies in SRO hotels or emergency shelters may not be applicable to the homeless who live in outdoor sites, or who live temporarily in the homes of family or friends (Roth & Bean, 1986).

Further, it is difficult to describe the health of the entire homeless population accurately because many homeless individuals resist interviews or do not seek care (Hingdon, 1984; Stoner, 1984). Many health studies on the homeless have only looked at those who sought medical care, who may not be representative of the population as a whole.

As a result of these and other important methodological differences, descriptions of the homeless vary significantly from study to study. Therefore, to describe the health of the homeless, this chapter focuses on trends that occur across studies despite differing methodologies and limited generalizability.

PHYSICAL ILLNESS

In comparison with the general population, the homeless have higher prevalence rates of physical morbidity (Alperstein, Rappaport, & Flanigan, 1988; Alstrom, Lindelius, & Salum, 1975; Cohen, 1988; Wright, Rossi, Knight, et al., 1985; Wright, Weber-Burdin, Knight, & Lam, 1987; Wright et al., 1987) as well as mortality. Reflecting this greater prevalence of illness, the homeless have poorer perceptions of their own health status than does the non-homeless population. One study, for example, found that 39% of homeless men compared with 21% of household men reported that they were in poor health (Fischer, Shapiro, Breaky, et al., 1986). Homeless adults most likely to have poor perceived health are those who have chronic physical illnesses, depression, and alcoholism (Ropers & Boyer, 1987). Similarly, homeless parents report low ratings for their children's health (Miller & Linn, 1988).

Physical illness appears to be taking its toll on the homeless and may be contributing to their inability to escape from homelessness; one quarter of homeless adults report that their health prevented them from working or going to school (Robertson and Cousineau, 1986; Rossi et al., 1987).

At least one third of homeless adults (Bassuk, Rubin, & Lauriat, 1986; Morse & Calsyn, 1986; Roth & Bean, 1986) and nearly one half of homeless children (Miller & Linn, 1988) report having a physical health problem. The primary medical diagnoses of homeless adults are related to upper-respiratory-tract infections, trauma, female genitourinary problems, hypertension, skin diseases, gastrointestinal disorders, and peripheral vascular diseases (Borg, 1978; Kelly &

Goldfinger, 1984; Rueler, Max, & Sampson, 1986; Wright et al., 1985; Wright, et al., 1987). One screening study found that at least one fourth of homeless adults had hypertension (Kellogg, Piantieri, Conanan, et al., 1984).

The primary medical difficulties of homeless children involve upper-respiratory-tract infections, skin diseases, ear diseases, dental problems, poor vision, gastrointestinal diseases, or trauma (Miller & Linn, 1988; Wood, Valdez, Hayashi, et al., 1989; Wright, et al., 1987). Homeless children are at least twice as likely to have these illnesses as children with homes (Wright, Weber-Burdin, Knight, & Lam, 1987).

As for obstetrical needs, Wright, Weber-Burdin, Knight, and Lam (1987), reported that 11% of homeless adult female patients and 24% of homeless female patients between 16 and 19 years old were pregnant. A comparative study (Chavkin, Kristal, Seabron, et al., 1987) of pregnancy among women of New York's hotels for the homeless, low-income housing projects, and other citywide dwellings found that women in hotels are more likely than other low-income women to have inadequate prenatal care (56%), a low-birthweight infant (16%), and a higher infant mortality rate (25 deaths/1,000 live births).

Research on contagious diseases among homeless persons has found that the homeless are more likely than the general population to have tuberculosis (McAdam, Brickner, Glicksman et al., 1985; Wright et al., 1985; Wright, Weber-Burdin, Knight, & Lam, 1987), and are difficult to treat because most have multiresistant organisms (Bernardo, Brigandi, Blakeney, et al., 1985). Among New York City's SRO residents, 51% had a positive tuberculosis skin test. Seven percent of the sample were subsequently found to have active tuberculosis (Sherman, Brickner, Schwartz, et al., 1980).

Researchers are also concerned about the spread of the acquired immunodeficiency syndrome (AIDS) among the homeless population. Torres, Lefkowitz, Kales, et al. (1987) reported that a high proportion (13%) of hospitalized AIDS patients were homeless; their main risk factor for AIDS was intravenous drug abuse. This suggests that the prevention, diagnosis, and treatment of infectious diseases among homeless populations will need to be addressed by health care, housing, and social service providers.

The homeless also have major problems with their dental health. One U.S. study reported that 10% of homeless adults had poor dentition, a rate 31 times that found in the general population (Wright,

Weber-Burdin, Knight, & Lam, 1987). A community-based survey in Los Angeles (Gelberg, Linn, & Leake, 1988) found that homeless adults were twice as likely as domiciled adults to have gross dental decay (57% versus 23%) but one third as likely to have obtained dental care in the past year. Given this high rate of dental disease, dental care should be an integral part of any health care service package developed for the homeless.

MENTAL ILLNESS

The media has made the public aware of the high prevalence of mental illness among the homeless and their desperate need for effective mental health treatment. Estimates of the prevalence of mental illness among homeless adults differ dramatically from study to study and range from 16% (Wright et al., 1985) to 91% (Bassuk, Rubin, & Lauriat, 1984). This wide range of estimates of mental illness may result from variations in populations sampled and the definition of mental illness used (Bachrach, 1987).

Despite the difficulty in comparing studies, empirical findings suggest that homeless adults are more than twice as likely as the general population to be mentally ill (Farr et al., 1986; Fischer et al., 1986). At least one third of homeless adults have a chronic serious psychiatric disorder including schizophrenia, affective disorders, and cognitive impairment (Farr et al., 1986). From 15% to 31% have a substance abuse disorder (Arce, Tadlock, Vergare, et al., 1983; Bassuk et al., 1984; Farr et al., 1986; Fischer et al., 1986; Sacks, Phillips, & Cappelletty, 1987). About 12% have dual diagnoses of chronic mental illness and chronic substance use (Farr et al., 1986; Wright, Weber-Burdin, Knight, & Lam, 1987). These latter individuals pose a challenge to developing services that will successfully address both aspects of their illness.

A similarly high prevalence of mental problems has been found among homeless children. Studies have found developmental delays in 25% to 47% of children younger than 5 years of age and depression in 31% of those older than 5 years of age (Bassuk et al., 1986; Wood, Valdez, et al., 1989). One study found that aggressive behavior problems were commoner in homeless children compared with housed poor children (Wood, Valdez, et al., 1989b). Development and mental health problems among homeless children are closely connected to the degree of dysfunction in the nuclear family, as evidenced by parental drug abuse, mental illness, or family violence (Wood, Hayashi, Schlossman, et al., 1989).

Because of the high prevalence of mental illness, the homeless are more likely than the general population to have been hospitalized for psychiatric care (Wright et al., 1987); from 15% to 44% of homeless adults have had a previous psychiatric hospitalization (Arce et al., 1983; Bassuk et al., 1984; Farr et al., 1986; Gelberg, Linn, & Leake, 1988; Kroll, Carey, Hagedorn, et al., 1986; Morse & Calsyn, 1986; Rossi et al., 1987; Roth & Bean, 1986; Segal, Baumohl, & Johnson, 1977; Susser, Struening, & Conover, 1987). Of these, 19% were hospitalized within the previous year (Fischer et al., 1986; Gelberg & Linn, 1988; Robertson et al., 1985). Although many of these previously hospitalized individuals had been hospitalized an average of five times in their lifetime, a significant subgroup (38%) had been hospitalized only once in their lifetime (Robertson et al., 1985), indicating that their mental illness may not be chronic. Alternatively, this group may reflect the current emphasis on outpatient rather than inpatient mental health treatment.

Despite their high prevalence of current mental illness, the homeless population has limited access to the outpatient mental health system (Fischer et al., 1986; Robertson et al., 1985).

EXPOSURE TO MORE RISK
FACTORS FOR ILLNESS

Homeless persons have higher rates of disease partially because disabling mental and physical illness may precipitate homelessness. Homelessness, and its attendant lifestyle and exposures, also are risk factors for disease, however. For instance, one study found that 41% of homeless adults reported that their health had become worse since becoming homeless (Robertson et al., 1984).

Homelessness may impact on the health of individuals through several aspects of the homeless life-style. Those who live outdoors in adverse weather conditions are susceptible to sunburn (17% were seriously sunburned in one Los Angeles study (Gelberg & Linn, 1988), dehydration, frostbite, and hypothermia (Brickner, Scharer, Conanan, et al., 1985; Lander, 1983). Moreover, homeless individuals experience physical and psychological trauma from victimization by robbery, beating, or sexual assault; in a given year, 37% of homeless adults had been injured and, on the average, victimized at least twice (Gelberg & Linn, 1988). Similarly, the homeless may develop burns if they sleep on hot grates, near steam vents, or near fires to keep warm; many have diseased feet from having poorly fitted shoes or having nowhere to elevate the legs (Wright et al., 1985). Because the quality and frequency of their meals are unpredictable, the homeless are thought to be at risk for malnutrition, obesity, hepatitis, and food poisoning (Beck & Marden, 1971).

The crowded living conditions of those who reside in shelters, and the often unsanitary living conditions of those who reside outdoors, may increase the risk of contagious diseases such as lice, scabies, impetigo, gastrointestinal infections, and respiratory-tract infections (Wright et al., 1985). Outbreaks of contagious diseases have been documented among the homeless in several communities including meningococcal disease in the skid rows of the Northwest (Filice, Englender, Jacobson, et al., 1984), pneumococcal pneumonia in a Boston shelter (DeMaria, Browne, Berk, et al., 1980), tuberculosis in Boston shelters (Barry, Wall, Shirley, Bernardo, et al., 1986; Bernardo et al., 1985; Nardell, McInnis, Thomas, et al., 1986), and diphtheria in both an Omaha mission (Heath & Zusman, 1962) and in Seattle's skid row (Pedersen, Spearman, Tonca, et al., 1977).

Finally, the homeless are at increased risk for most diseases because of their high prevalence of adverse health habits such as cigarette smoking, alcoholism (Cohen, 1988; Borg, 1978; Rossi et al., 1987b; Wright, Weber-Burdin, Knight, et al., 1987), and drug abuse (Wright, Weber-Burdin, Knight, & Lam, 1987; Wright, Weber-Burdin, Geronimo, 1987). A broad-based survey of the homeless in Los Angeles (Robertson et al., 1985) found that 64% were currently using alcohol, and 55% had used at least one illicit drug more than five times in their lifetime; one third of those who had used drugs reported feelings of dependency on at least one drug.

BARRIERS TO CARE

Homeless adults are less likely than the general adult population to use outpatient medical services (Fischer et al., 1986) but more likely to be hospitalized (often for a preventable condition) (Cohen, 1988; Fischer et al., 1986; Kelly & Goldfinger, 1984; Robertson et al.,

1985). This indicates that the homeless encounter major obstacles to obtaining needed medical and psychiatric services. Most homeless adults state that they did not obtain needed medical care in the previous year (Gelberg & Linn, 1988; Robertson & Cousineau, 1986). Even among those with a chronic medical condition, one half had not seen a doctor within the previous year (Robertson et al., 1985).

The homeless confront numerous problems in obtaining appropriate health care. First, they face financial barriers. One fifth cited lack of money as the primary reason they had not obtained needed medical care in the previous year (Cohen, 1988). Most of the homeless have no public or private health insurance (Bassuk et al., 1984; Farr et al., 1986; Miller & Lin, 1988; Robertson et al., 1985). Complicated application and eligibility requirements keep many homeless from obtaining health insurance and other services for which they are eligible. For example, they may not have an identification card, a record of their work history and medical treatment history, or a stable address to receive correspondence from social service agencies (Segal et al., 1977).

Second, transportation to medical facilities is often unavailable to this population (Robertson & Cousineau, 1986). In many parts of the country, the homeless must take several buses and travel 2 to 3 hours to the nearest medical facility providing health care to indigents. As detailed in this book, health services would be more effective if they were located in accessible locations where the homeless tend to visit and live such as shelters, soup lines, or outdoor congregation areas (Sacks et al., 1987).

Third, homeless persons with disabling mental illness, although in great need of health services, are often unable to obtain them. One study found that psychological distress among homeless adults was positively related to not having obtained needed care during the previous year (Gelberg & Linn, 1989). For example, Bassuk et al. (1984) found that only 4 of 30 acutely psychotic homeless patients in their shelter study took psychotropic medications. Paranoia, lack of social supports, disorientation, and lack of organizational skills to gain access to needed services (Bachrach, 1987), or a fear of institutions and authority figures resulting from previous institutionalization (Cohen & Dronska, 1988) keep many homeless persons from obtaining psychiatric help.

Fourth, traditional mental health services may not be appropriate to meet the needs of this population. Homeless mentally ill individuals are often wary of traditional mental health services

(Bachrach, 1987). One St. Louis study, for example, found that 73% of the mentally ill homeless were willing to receive mental health care but not in a traditional mental health setting. Mental health services provided through residential services, day programs, or case management were found more acceptable (Morse & Calsyn, 1986). This may be because traditional services cannot handle their multifaceted problems, which include not only mental illness, but substance abuse, physical illness, criminal behavior, and extreme social isolation (Crystal, 1984; Gelberg & Linn, 1988; Gelberg et al., 1988; Morse & Calsyn, 1986).

Fifth, the homeless may sense that the medical profession itself imposes barriers to care. Some medical providers consider the homeless to be undesirable patients because of their poor hygiene and mental illness, or because of assumptions that they come to hospitals for shelter and not for a medical problem (Baxter & Hopper, 1981).

Sixth, street life may affect compliance with medical care. The homeless often lack a place to keep medications safe, intact, and refrigerated, and are unable to obtain the proper food for a medically indicated diet (Brickner et al., 1985; Wright et al., 1985). In addition, many homeless individuals may be so transient that they are unlikely to maintain the follow-up and continuity of care that is so important to the management of chronic illness (Brickner et al., 1984; Wright et al., 1985).

CONCLUSION

In summary, the homeless face an overwhelming set of physical, dental, mental, and social problems. They suffer from more illness and are more likely to be hospitalized for medical and psychiatric problems than the general population. Given the extent of illness in this population, however, the homeless are less likely than the general population to use outpatient medical services. This indicates that homeless individuals experience significant barriers to obtaining medical care.

Thus, the data suggest that more effective health services need to be developed for the homeless population. The following chapters will provide detailed and practical descriptions of how to provide health care to homeless persons that is tailored to their special needs, priorities, and health problems.

REFERENCES

Alperstein, G., Rappaport, C., & Flanigan J. M. (1988). Health problems of homeless children in New York City. *American Journal of Public Health, 78,* 1232–1233.

Alstrom, C. H., Lindelius, R., Salum, I. (1975). Mortality among homeless men. *British Journal of Addiction, 70,* 245–252.

Arce, A. A., Tadlock, M., Vergare, M. J., et al. (1983). A psychiatric profile of street people admitted to an emergency shelter. *Hospital Community Psychiatry, 34,* 812–817.

Bachrach, L. L. (1987). Issues in identifying and treating the homeless mentally ill. In R. H. Lamb (Ed.), *New directions for mental health services* (pp. 43–62). San Francisco: Jossey-Bass.

Barry, M. A., Wall, C., Shirley, L., Bernardo, J., et al. (1986). Tuberculosis screening in Boston's homeless shelters. *Public Health Report, 101,* 487–494.

Bassuk, E. L., Rubin, L., Lauriat, A. (1984). Is homelessness a mental health problem? *American Journal of Psychology, 141,* 1546–1550.

Bassuk, E. L., Rubin, L., & Lauriat, A. (1986). Characteristics of sheltered homeless families. *American Journal of Public Health, 76,* 1097–1101.

Baxter, E. K., & Hopper, (1981). *Private lives/public spaces: Homeless adults on the streets of New York.* New York: Community Service Society, Institute for Social Welfare Research.

Beck, A. M., & Marden, P. (1971). Street dwellers. *Natural History, 86,* 78–85.

Bernardo, J., Brigandi, E., Blakeney, B., et al. (1985). Drug-resistant tuberculosis among the homeless. *Morbidity and Morality Weekly Report, 34,* 429–431.

Borg, S. (1978). Homeless men: *A clinical and social study with special reference to alcohol abuse.* Munksgaard, Copenhagen: Institute Department of Psychiatry.

Brickner, P. W., Scharer, L. K., Conanan, B., et al. (1985). *Health care of homeless people.* New York: Springer.

Chavkin, W., Kristal, A., Seabron, C., et al. (1987). The reproductive experience of women living in hotels for the homeless in New York City. *New York State Journal of Medicine, 87*(1), 10–13.

Cohen, C. (1988). Survival strategies of older homeless men. *Journal of Gerontology, 28,* 58–65.

Cohen, M. A., & Dronska. H. (1988). Treatment refusal in a rootless individual with medical problems. *General Hospital Psychiatry, 10,* 61–66.

Crystal, S. (1984). Homeless men and homeless women: The gender gap. *Urban Sociology Change Revew, 17,* 2–6.

DeMaria, A, Browne, K., Berk, S. L., et al. (1980). An outbreak of type 1 pneumococcal pneumonia in a men's shelter. *Journal of the American Medical Association, 244*, 1446–1449.

Farr, R. K., Koegel, P., & Burnam, A. (1986, March). *A Study of homelessness and mental illness in the skid row area of Los Angeles*. Los Angeles County; Department of Mental Health.

Filice, G. A., Englender, S. J., Jacobson, J. A., et al. (1984). Group A meningococcal disease in skid rows: Epidemiology and implications for control. *Public Health Briefs, 74*, 253–254.

Fischer, P. J., & Breaky, W. R. (1987). Profile of the Baltimore homeless with alcohol problems. *Alcohol Health and Research World, 11*, 36–37, 61.

Fischer, P. J., Shapiro, S., Breaky, W. R., et al. (1986). Mental health and social characteristics of the homeless: A survey of mission users. *American Journal of Public Health, 76*, 669–678.

Gelberg, L., & Linn, L. (1988). Users of mental health services: A portrait of homeless adults. *Hospital Community Psychiatry, 39*, 510–516.

Gelberg, L., Linn, L., & Leake, B. D. (1988). Mental health, alcohol and drug use, and criminal history among homeless adults. *American Journal of Psychiatry, 145*, 191–196.

Gelberg, L., Linn, L. S., & Rosenberg, D. J. (1988). Dental health of homeless adults. *Special Care Dentistry, 8*, 167–172.

Heath, C. W., & Zusman, J. (1962). An outbreak of diphtheria among skid-row men. *New England Journal of Medicine, 267*, 809–812.

Hingdon, L. (1984). *The homeless poor, 1984—Multnomah County, Oregon*. Multnomah County: Oregon Department of Health and Human Services, Social Services Division.

Hombs, M. E., & Snyder, M. (1982). *Homelessness in America: A forced march to nowhere*. Washington, DC: Community for Creative Nonviolence.

Kellogg, F. R., Piantieri, O., Conanan, B., et al. (1984). *A hypertension screening and treatment program for the homeless*. New York: St. Vincent's Hospital and Medical Center of New York.

Kelly, J. T., & Goldfinger, S. M. (1984). *Hospitalization of the homeless: An analysis*. San Francisco: University of California.

Kroll, J., Carey, K., Hagedorn, D., et al. (1986). A survey of homeless adults in urban emergency shelters. *Hospital Community Psychiatry, 37*, 283–286.

Lander, R. (1983, February 23). *Health needs of the homeless: An overview* [Transcript of a lecture presented to the Coalition's Providers' Caucus]. New York: Coalition for the Homeless.

Levine, I. S. (1984). Homelessness implications for mental health policy and practice. *Psychosocial Rehabilitation Journal, 8*, 6–16.

McAdam, J., Brickner, P. W., Glicksman, R., et al. (1985). Tuberculosis in the SRO/homeless population. In Brickner P. W. et al. (Eds.), *Health care of homeless people*. New York: Springer.

Miller, D. S., & Lin, E. H. B. (1988). Children in sheltered homeless families: Reported health status and utilization of health services. *Pediatrics, 81,* 668–673.

Morse, G., & Calsyn. R. J. (1986). Mentally disturbed homeless people in St. Louis: Needy, willing, but underserved. *International Journal of Mental Health, 14,* 74–94.

Nardell, E., McInnis, B., Thomas, B., et al. (1986). Exogenous reinfection with tuberculosis in a shelter for the homeless. *New England Journal of Medicine, 315,* 1570–1575.

Pedersen, A. H. B., Spearman, J., Tonca, E., et al. (1977). Diphtheria on skid road, Seattle, Washington, 1972–75. *Public Health Report, 92,* 336–342.

Robertson, M. J., & Cousineau, M. R. (1986). Health status and access to health services among the urban homeless. *American Journal of Public Health, 76,* 561–563.

Robertson, M. J., Ropers, R. H., & Boyer, R. (1984). *Emergency shelter for the homeless in Los Angeles County.* Los Angeles: UCLA School of Public Health.

Robertson, M. J., Ropers, R. H., & Boyer, R. (1985). *The homeless of Los Angeles County: An empirical evaluation.* Los Angeles: UCLA Basic Shelter Research Project.

Ropers, R. H., & Boyer, R. (1987). Perceived health status among the new urban homeless. *Social Science and Medicine, 24,* 669–678.

Rossi, P. H., Wright, J. D., Fisher, G. A., et al. (1987). The urban homeless: Estimating composition and size. *Science, 235,* 1336–1341.

Roth, D., & Bean, J. (1986). New perspective on homelessness: Findings from a statewide epidemiological study. *Hospital Community Psychiatry, 37,* 712–719.

Rueler, J. B., Max, M. J., & Sampson, J. H. (1986). Physician house call services for medically needy inner-city residents. *American Journal of Public Health, 76,* 1131–1134.

Sacks, J. M., Phillips, J., & Cappelletty, G. (1987). Characteristics of the homeless mentally disordered population in Fresno County. *Community Mental Health Journal, 23,* 114–119.

Segal, S. P., Baumohl, J., & Johnson, E. (1977). Falling through the cracks: Mental disorder and social margin in a young vagrant population. *Social Problems, 24,* 387–401.

Sherman, M. N., Brickner, P. W., Schwartz, M. S., et al. (1980, Fall). Tuberculosis in single-room-occupancy hotel residents: A persisting focus of disease. *New York Medical Quarterly,* 39–41.

Stoner, M. R. (1984). An analysis of public and private sector provisions for homeless people. *Urban Social Change Review, 17,* 3–8.

Susser, E., Struening, E. L., & Conover, S. (1987). Childhood experiences of homeless men. *American Journal of Psychiatry, 144,* 1599–1601.

Torres, R. A., Lefkowitz, P., Kales, C., et al. (1987). Homelessness among hospitalized patients with the acquired immunodeficiency syndrome in New York City. *Journal of the American Medical Association, 258,* 779–780.

Wood, D., Hayashi, T., Schlossman, S., et al. (1989, August). Over the brink: Homeless families in Los Angeles. Sacramento: Assembly Office of Research.

Wood, D., Valdez, R., Hayashi, T., et al. (in press). The health of homeless children. *Pediatrics.*

Wright, J. D., Rossi, P. H., Knight, J. W., et al. (1985, January). *Health and homelessness in New York City.* Amherst: University of Massachusetts, The Social and Demographic Research Institute.

Wright, J. D., Rossi, P. H., Knight, J. W., Weber-Burdin, E., Tessler, R. C., Stewart, C. E., Geronimo, M., & Lam, J. (1987). Homelessness and health: The effects of life style on physical well-being among homeless people in New York City. *Research on Social Problems and Public Policy, 4,* 41–72.

Wright, J. D., Weber-Burdin, E., Geronimo, M., et al. (1987). Homelessness and health. *Research on Social Problems and Public Policy.*

Wright, J. D., Weber-Burdin, E., Knight, J. W., Lam, J. A. (1987, March). The National Health Care for the Homeless Program: The first year. Amherst: University of Massachusetts, The Social and Demographic Research Institute.

Wright, J. D., Weber-Burdin, E., Knight, J. W., et al. (1987). Ailments and alcohol: Health status among the drinking homeless. *Alcohol Health and Research World, 11,* 22–27.

Patient-Oriented Approach to Providing Care to Homeless Persons

2

Paul Koegel, Lillian Gelberg

CHAPTER HIGHLIGHTS

- Three fictional case studies are presented to emphasize the special needs of homeless persons: a 29-year-old homeless man with newly diagnosed diabetes; a schizophrenic with a badly infected hand; and a 12-year-old homeless boy who is frightened and having learning problems.
- The homeless environment and the attitudes and beliefs of homeless individuals influence their decision to seek medical care and their behavior in the health care center.
- The homeless have no access to beds in which to convalesce, have little control over what or when they eat, cannot refrigerate their medication, are often unable to maintain adequate hygiene, and, to ensure that their survival needs are met, must frantically juggle the schedules of several service programs.
- Because the homeless have little or no financial resources, any medical regimen that requires money for care or medications is problematic.
- The mobility of homeless patients makes continuity of care difficult.
- The attitudes of homeless people toward services, their priorities, and their view of time may differ from those of providers, setting up the possibility of conflict and failure of communication or treatment.

INTRODUCTION

Imagine that a new university clinic has been constructed 3 miles from the center of a large city, where the area's largest concentration of homeless individuals resides. No expense has been spared in designing this facility; it is modern, clean, and well staffed. Its doors open up with much fanfare—speeches by politicians, ribbon cutting, media coverage—and staff settles in to await their first patients, who are not long in arriving.

Meanwhile, in the inner city, Joe, 29 years old and a relatively new arrival to the ranks of the homeless, is managing to survive. Two months earlier, he had left his home in Alabama when his family, struggling to make ends meet, made it clear that they could no longer provide housing for him. Joe had packed his bags, pocketed the $500 he scraped together to tide him over until he could get a job, and headed for the city, where he figured the opportunities would be better. Two days later, shortly after arriving at the city's Greyhound Bus Terminal late at night, he was "rolled," losing all he had. Ashamed at being in such dire straits so soon after leaving home and convinced that his family did not have the resources to help him anyway, he made no attempt to contact them for help. Joe spent that first night sitting outside the bus terminal but within a relatively brief period, learned the ropes so that this was no longer necessary. Two months later, he was well entrenched in a subsistence pattern that allowed him to meet his basic needs but that left him time for little else.

For instance, Joe spent the previous night in the Green Street shelter. Because breakfast at the shelter is restricted to women and handicapped individuals, Joe goes to the Rescue Mission at 6:30 a.m. where he stands in line to enter the chapel, sits through mandatory services, and then eats. The mission has facilities for showering and laundering clothes, and because Joe's appearance remains important to him, he takes advantage of them. Lines are long, however, and it is not until 9:30 a.m. that he leaves the mission.

As early as it is, Joe turns his attention to lunch, knowing that another long wait in line will be necessary. It is a long walk from the Rescue Mission to a local soup kitchen, but the food is appreciably better there. Joe makes the trek across town, arriving at 10:30 a.m. Even at that early hour, his place in line is well to the rear. The doors open at 11:00 a.m., but Joe is not served until 11:30 a.m. Because he wants seconds, he has to enter the line again, and it is not until 12:30

p.m. that he is finished. From there, it is back to the Rescue Mission in the hopes of securing a bed for the night, because the policy at the Green Street Shelter is "1 night out, 1 night in." A lottery is held for the available bed tickets at the Rescue Mission, and Joe is lucky. He will have shelter for the next week, because this facility's policy is "7 days in, 5 days out." Had he not secured a bed, his remaining option would have been to sit up in a chair in the chapel all night, which leaves him stiff and causes his legs to swell. Joe leaves the Rescue Mission at 3:00 p.m. for another facility, where dinner tickets are being distributed. He secures one after another long wait, hangs out for a while in their reading room, queues up for the meal, and then returns to the Rescue Mission by 7:00 p.m. for his bed.

As preoccupied as Joe has been with this new schedule, he has been unable to ignore the fact that something is physically wrong with him. He has been urinating more than usual, a real problem given his difficulty in accessing bathrooms. He has also been feeling thirsty despite drinking a lot of water and more hungry than usual, even though he is getting enough food. In addition, he has been bothered by a growth on his foot, which he attributes to all the walking he has been doing.

Joe has heard of the new university clinic—posters have been prominently displayed in many city facilities—but it has been difficult to figure out how he will get there. Taking the bus is out of the question, because Joe has no money and finds panhandling distasteful. An hour-long walk each way is the only alternative. This may mean forfeiting lunch and not getting back to the mission in time to claim his bed. For these reasons, he has been putting it off. He has become increasingly concerned, however, because the symptoms have been intensifying. He finally decides to set out for the new clinic after his morning shower, hoping that he will be back in time for dinner.

Joe's reception at the clinic is distant and suspicious as they notice his clothing, which is neat but not as stylish or as well coordinated as that worn by the clinic's regular clientele. The receptionist asks to see his health insurance card, and he explains that he does not have one. She is about to refuse him care and direct him to the public health facilities when Joe passes out in the reception room. As Joe wakes up, he finds a nurse taking his vital signs; she brings him into a room. Joe must wait a long time to be seen by the physician because the clinic patients are mostly there by appointment, and, despite the fact that he feels quite sick, his condition does not seem to the clinic staff to warrant an emergency response. Several frustrating hours later, he is finally screened by a nurse practitioner and seen by a doctor, who performs a thorough examination including blood work and urinalysis. The news is not good. Ketones in his urine and a high blood sugar confirm the physician's suspicions of diabetes, and suggest an advanced enough case to require the injection of insulin. The nurse will teach him how to inject himself, the doctor explains, and will tell him more about the care and refrigeration of his insulin supply. Joe says nothing.

Joe's problems, however, go beyond diabetes. His legs, it seems, show signs of pedal edema because of venous stasis—swelling from not lying down—that places him at risk for leg ulcers and possibly a life-threatening infection. The doctor advises him to elevate his feet whenever he sits or lies down, using another chair or pillows to do so. The doctor also states that the growth on the bottom of Joe's foot should be removed. She reassures him that it is a minor procedure that can be performed in the office but that it will have to be performed at the public clinic where they see more poor people. Furthermore, Joe is told to bring someone along to drive him home if he lives too far away to navigate the distance on crutches. Jokingly, she tells him that unless he is a champion hopper, he will probably need some help looking after himself for a day or two. Finally, as a matter of course she gives him a PPD (purified protein derivative) test, explaining that it is a skin examination for tuberculosis, and tells him to come back to the clinic in 2 or 3 days to get the results.

The interaction is over and the doctor gone before Joe has mustered the courage to swallow his pride and confess that he is homeless, and that the doctor's advice is thus problematic. Outside in the reception area, he evaluates his position. There is no chance of refrigerating insulin, in that he has no access to a refrigerator. Furthermore, Joe is extremely apprehensive about possessing clean hypodermics, fearing that they will make him the target of intravenous drug users, who heavily prize such items.

The suggestion that he stay off his feet is completely out of the question in that his survival depends on his ability to move from place to place. He is not sure that there is anyone he can ask to accompany him to the clinic for the minor surgery; nor does he know anyone with transportation or the means to care for him for several days. Moreover, the clinic obviously is not interested in his problems because it does not want to see him again, so it probably does not matter if he gets the PPD test read, a task that would require walking the 3 miles again. His lungs feel fine, which he hopes means that the test would be negative anyway.

All in all, he feels more depressed than he did before coming to the clinic. He now knows what is wrong with him but feels unable to do anything about it. In addition, he bears the unwanted burden of knowing he has medical problems, the solutions to which seem out of reach.

As he makes his way back to the inner city, Joe passes a disheveled man who regularly sits on the same corner, talking aloud in an agitated fashion. Joe has seen him many times. His clothes are tattered and filthy, he reeks of sweat and urine, and he gives every indication of being crazy. Walking by, Joe thinks to himself that he should count his blessings. There are those who are worse off than he.

Frank, the man Joe passes, is schizophrenic. Discharged from the army 5 years ago when he began hearing voices and behaving strangely, he had managed to get a menial job working in a hotel, where he was also able to live. As his behavior became more erratic, he was fired. Frank temporarily joined the Job Corps but began suspecting that those around him were part of a Central Intelligence Agency design to kill him. For his own safety, he left the program. Having no income, he began living under a freeway overpass, which has been his home for the last several years.

Frank spends his days on the same street corner. Wary of crowds and fiercely independent, he scavenges and relies on unsolicited handouts for his food, entering service facilities only when hunger compels him to or cold weather forces him to spend the night in the mission chapel chairs. Periodically, his existence has been interrupted by the unwanted intervention of the police or a psychiatric emergency team. His stays in crowded psychiatric wards, each resulting in discharge to the streets, have only made him determined to avoid such encounters.

While scavenging in a dumpster a week ago, Frank cut his hand on the lid of a can. This is not the first time something like this has happened, but this time the hand has not healed. Before long, the wound is oozing pus, and the pain and swelling are considerable, making it difficult for Frank to ignore it. Like Joe, he knows about the university clinic. As much as he hates doctors and medical settings, he decides to seek care. Leaving his corner, he navigates the long walk to the clinic. Its modern facade, large size, and the conspicuous presence of a uniformed guard by the entrance, however, combine to spook him. Aware of how out of place he is and wildly anxious about entering, he turns and leaves.

The hand worsens, however, and several days later Frank tries again. This time, he forces himself through the door and into the reception area, where the receptionist views him with alarm and those in the waiting room pull away, increasing his intense anxiety and making it more difficult to ignore the voices in his head telling him to leave. Because of his stench and his refusal to leave, he is shown almost immediately to a small, antiseptic examination room, which sparks intense feelings of claustrophobia. He is becoming extremely agitated, a condition that is not eased by the entering physician, whose white coat reminds him all too well of psychiatric personnel. He manages to contain himself as the doctor cleans and examines his wound, and he accepts the prescription for antibiotics and a pain killer. He asks no questions as the doctor informs him that he can fill the prescriptions at the clinic pharmacy, instructs him to take the pain medication with meals, and advises him to change the dressing regularly and keep it clean. When the doctor volunteers that he is concerned about Frank's mental health and wonders whether he has been hearing voices, however, Frank is sure that another stay in the county hospital is imminent. He bolts out of the room and back to the streets where he is free, even if in pain.

Eying Frank's mad dash through the waiting room with some curiousity is Robert, who at 12 years of age is the oldest of his 28-year-old mother's four children. It is Robert's 18-month-old sister, Kanisha, whose problems have brought them to the clinic. Shortly after they moved into the family shelter 2 weeks ago, Kanisha developed diarrhea and a high fever that have shown no signs of abating. Robert hates the shelter, where all the babies seem to scream as loud as Kanisha. They live on cots amid countless other families, and his mother's temper has been exceptionally short lately. Life had been just as bad, though, when they were living with his mother's drug-abusing boyfriend. The family was evicted from their apartment when the boyfriend used some of the rent money for drugs. They then went to live with Robert's grandmother. It was much better there despite the overcrowding; three families, including four adults and seven children were crammed into a small two-bedroom house. After several months, tensions rose and culminated in the argument that led to their leaving. During these months, Robert's mother had actively looked for an apartment but could not find one she could afford that would accept their family with four children. Robert figured it was all Welfare's fault—if they had not been erroneously kicked off, his mother and grandmother probably would not have been fighting in the first place.

Robert is anxious as he sits in the waiting room with his family. Actually, he and his siblings have been anxious a lot lately. One of his younger brothers has started wetting the bed again even though he has long since been toilet trained. Robert is particularly anxious because he knows that tomorrow he will have to enter a new school, his fifth school in 2 years. He misses his friends from his old neighborhood and is tired of making new friends. He knows the other children at the school will make fun of him for wearing secondhand cloths and living at the shelter. He is also discouraged because his performance at school is getting worse and worse; he gets nothing but negative feedback from the teacher, and, for the first time in his life, he suspects that he may be really stupid.

Robert's anxiety is exacerbated today, however, because he is afraid of what will happen when they see the doctor. He knows that they are there because Kanisha is sick but wonders what else the doctor will ask. Will he be able to recognize that even though his brother looks OK now, he sometimes wheezes and cannot breathe? Will he yell at Robert for not going to school regularly? Will he notice the bruises on his arms from where his mother's boyfriend grabbed him and shook him, which he would like to talk about but is afraid to? Will the doctor take him and his siblings away from their mother as had happened to another child at the shelter, even though she loves them and takes pretty good care of them (at least most of the time)? Robert is not sure what to hope for: He wants the doctor to help them but does not want the doctor to get them in trouble.

Robert feels frightened as he and his family are called into the examination room. Robert soon realizes, however, that the doctor is paying attention to no one but Kanisha and her relatively mild symptoms. The doctor explains to his mother that Kanisha has an intestinal infection and that it is very important for her to drink clear liquids and electrolyte solutions. For the fever, the doctor prescribes acetaminophen and tepid baths. His mother is quiet, and Robert knows she is wondering how this will be possible in the shelter, where bathroom time is at a premium and where there are only showers. He listens as the doctor tells his mother that once the diarrhea dissipates, Kanisha should slowly be introduced to bananas, rice, applesauce, and toast, and that dairy products should be avoided. That confuses Robert, because they eat only what they are given at the shelter, having no money to buy anything else. Still, the fact that the doctor has given his mother some acetaminophen reassures Robert. Though none of their other problems have been addressed, perhaps the medicine will help.

The experiences of Joe, Frank, and Robert—three extremely different people—all highlight the fact that delivery of health care to homeless people will be neither successful nor comprehensive unless it is sensitive to the special circumstance of those living without homes and to the attitudes of homeless people. Having emphasized (by example) how heterogeneous this population is, we would be hard-pressed to argue that there is one formula that can govern the provision of services to all homeless people. We do believe, however, that when health care for the homeless is guided by a uniquely patient-oriented approach—one that takes as its starting point an understanding of the concerns and life-styles of homeless people—the service-related interactions that follow will invariably result in more satisfying and productive interactions between practitioner and patient.

In what follows, we briefly introduce some of these issues and their importance to health service planners and clinicians. The issues we discuss are not meant to be exhaustive or relevant to every homeless subgroup. They will, however, begin to clarify how a patient-oriented approach can result in more effective health care for the homeless. Furthermore, the remaining chapters in this book will discuss in detail the application of the patient-oriented approach for specific health conditions and among particular homeless subpopulations.

HOMELESS LIFE-STYLES AND THEIR CONSEQUENCES FOR MEDICAL REGIMENS

Housing is such a basic need that few people ever think about how central a home is to everything they do. In the case of health practitioners, timeworn ways of dealing with patients and their problems are all based on the assumption that the individual has a home. It is thus essential that those delivering health care to homeless persons carefully consider how their usual procedures and advice will be heard and experienced by those who do not have a home.

Problems in Meeting Basic Needs

When one matches common medical procedure against the reality of a homeless existence, several implications of homelessness immediately become apparent. Perhaps most glaringly, homeless individuals lack access to places in which they can convalesce in bed. Most live either in shelters, to which they do not have access during daytime hours, or out on streets. Although some homeless people may have access to daytime beds in drop-in centers, these tend to be cots set up in crowded, noisy, and often smoky environments. Bed rest, to say the least, is problematic; keeping off one's feet is a near impossibility.

Meeting other basic needs is difficult as well. Largely dependent on soup kitchens and other meal programs, the homeless usually have little control over what or when they eat. Thus, regimens that rely on dietary changes or involve taking medications with meals are impractical. Likewise, most homeless people lack access to refrigerators—especially locked refrigerators—and will be unable to follow advice regarding refrigerating medication. Personal hygiene, too, can be a problem, especially among those who shy away from contact with service facilities. Even those who make use of available showers and bathrooms find it difficult to maintain adequate hygiene as competition is fierce for these scarce resources. Infection prevention strategies that center on repeated applications of soap and hot running water may thus be extremely difficult to implement.

Though we typically think of homeless people as having an inordinate amount of time on their hands, often they must frantically juggle the schedules of several service settings to ensure that all their needs are met. The endless waits in line makes homelessness a full-time job for many. What is more, getting food or a bed for the night is often dependent on being in a certain place at a certain time. Failing to do so can mean forfeiting something essential to a homeless person's survival.

Storage is a major problem for homeless individuals. Most do not have access to closets and medicine cabinets, and thus must carry their possessions with them. Suggesting that someone use pillows to elevate a swollen foot or a pail to soak the foot may require that person to double the bulk he carries. The fact that homeless people must carry their possessions with them also means that the medication and paraphernalia required to treat their illness will, in all likelihood, be on their person at all times. This could make them targets for victimization as certain medications, especially those with recreational value or the needles required to inject them, are highly valued on the street.

Limited Financial Resources

Homeless people have so much trouble meeting their basic needs because they have little or no money. Some have no cash resources at all despite their eligibility for public entitlements. Any regimen that involves money may thus be problematic, no matter how small the cost. Limited financial resources may also affect access to health care facilities that are not centrally located and within easy walking distance. If getting medical care is too arduous, costly, or time-consuming, it may be postponed or completely avoided.

Limited Social Supports

Many homeless persons are further handicapped because they have few or no social supports, or because their social network members do not have resources to provide needed assistance. They often have no one who can transport them from a clinic or provide care for several days after an invasive procedure.

Mobility

Although most homeless individuals are long-term residents of their community, a significant minority of homeless travel extensively. Further, even those with long-standing ties to a given community display high intracity mobility because of their tenuous hold on subsistence resources. This mobility makes continuity of care difficult: An individual who is supposed to return to a clinic may not do so because he or she has moved; health care providers may not be able to recontact a homeless individual, even though test results reveal a life-threatening condition.

Multiple, Interwoven Problems of Homeless People

Homeless people are usually mired in myriad interconnected problems. Their presenting complaint may be the tip of an iceberg that includes other health, mental health, substance abuse, and daily living problems such as not having a place to stay, difficulties with the public assistance system, inability to keep ahead in school, lack of child care, or legal troubles. Homeless individuals may also experience extreme demoralization resulting from stress and constant assaults to their self-esteem. Among single adults, this may manifest itself in situational depression that seriously hampers their ability to follow medical advice. Among couples, homelessness leads to strained relationships, heightening the possibility of substance abuse and domestic violence. Children often react to insecurity and lack of nurturing with disruptive or withdrawn behavior, and may be at risk for any number of serious problems including developmental delay.

Health care providers must look beyond the presenting problem and be prepared to intervene on many fronts, some of which do not lie within the traditional boundaries of medicine. That some homeless people will not want, at least at first, to deal with anything other than the problem for which they are seeking care only complicates a difficult situation.

IMPACT OF ATTITUDES, VALUES, AND WORLD VIEWS

Culture plays a significant role in the delivery of health care: Differences in how practitioners and patients view illness, and in the expectations they bring to their relationship, can negatively affect the quality of medical care. Because the homeless population includes people from so many backgrounds, and because this group lacks the clear boundaries (like language or ethnic identity) that signal the potential importance of cultural sensitivity, health practitioners can all too easily ignore the possibility that cultural factors influence their relationships with homeless clients. This is unfortunate, because although it may be difficult to talk about a "culture" of homelessness to which all homeless individuals subscribe, it is reasonable to suggest that health care practitioners and their homeless clients may view health care–related matters very differently. The attitudes of homeless people toward services, their priorities, and their view of concepts such as time may differ from those of providers, setting up the possibility of conflict and failure.

Attitudes Toward Services

Many homeless individuals—especially those who have been homeless for a long time and those who suffer from chronic mental illness or substance abuse—may be alienated from mainstream society. Those who are leery of formal services may view an imposing edifice like the fictional university clinic described earlier as frightening, and may worry that they will be faced by unfamiliar rules and codes of behvaior if they enter. For some, such as Frank, these feelings may be powerful enough to impede their access. Even when homeless individuals (such as Joe or Robert's mother) are not alienated from formal services, embarrassment regarding their homeless condition may threaten a successful interaction. Many individuals will not admit they are homeless, creating the kind of misunderstanding that led Joe's physician to suggest procedures that he could not carry out. Also, some patients, although willing to admit to homelessness, may be embarrassed by factors related to their homeless condition. If, for instance, Joe had not had access to a shower and clean clothes, he might have resisted to disrobing for a thorough medical examination because he had been wearing the same pair of underpants for 2 months.

Priorities

The priorities of homeless patients and health care providers are often markedly different. Although practitioners view health care decisions from the logic of medical practice, homeless patients base decisions on a very different set of variables. No matter how life threatening, health problems may be dismissed as secondary to more immediate needs, such as a bed for the night or an evening meal. Unfortunately, this means that health practitioners must often deal with conditions that would have been far easier to treat had the individual sought help earlier.

In addition to delaying treatment, a homeless person may seek attention for one condition but show signs of other, more serious problems. Although from a medical viewpoint it may make sense to deal with the more serious condition first, this logic may contradict the equally rational logic underlying the patient's preference that the less serious condition be given immediate attention. Given the myraid problems they are experiencing, for instance, homeless individuals may assign primary importance to problems that are visible or that they can feel. Similarly, they may assign primacy to problems that are immediate in their consequences. An infected hand inhibits one's ability to survive on a daily basis; the threat of a heart attack 5 years in the future because of hypertension is simply too far off to be meaningful now. Lastly, they may not want to even know that they have maladies other than their presenting problem, because such information may overwhelm their ability to cope.

This situation poses a major dilemma for health care practitioners. Do they simply treat the problem about which the patient is concerned, or do they treat the patient's problems in the order suggested by good medical practice? Although there is no easy answer to this question, experience suggests that homeless individuals must feel that their priorities are being attended to—that they are being given what they think they need. Doing so may foster the rapport that will eventually allow the health care practitioner's agenda to be implemented.

Homeless persons may also turn to health care practitioners for help with basic needs such as food, shelter, clothing, and money that health care practitioners view as not falling within their bailiwick. We believe that these are legitimate areas of intervention for the health practitioner, if not directly then certainly by immediate referral and follow-through assistance. Such intervention, which can be thought of as prevention, fosters critically important rapport, thus increasing the likelihood that successful medical care will occur. It also addresses the unhealthful conditions that underlie the medical problems people are experiencing.

Attitude Toward Time

In addition to their attitude toward services and priorities, the mind-set of homeless people differs in more subtle ways from that of health practitioners. Take the concept of time, for example. Rather than viewing time as linear, as mainstream society does, people who have been homeless for long periods tend to see time as cyclical. Homeless people take their cues from the events that mark their daily and monthly cycles—the opening and closing of a shelter, the time at which meals or bed tickets are handed out, the arrival of a monthly check—and not as much by an arbitrary clock. Indeed, most homeless do not own or wear watches, primarily because they are so easily stolen.

Even formal service delivery systems end up subtly reinforcing this cyclical view of time. People who appear for a 10:00 a.m. appointment at the Social Security Administration, for instance, may not be seen for 2 hours. Indeed, one agency that serves homeless individuals in Los Angeles has given up any pretense of maintaining its own appointment schedule and now assigns people a day, rather than an hour, to meet with their eligibility worker. Homeless persons' more relaxed sense of time creates the possibility for misunderstanding when, for example, a health clinic for homeless individuals tries to maintain a fixed schedule.

In addition to viewing time as cyclical, the homeless, like other poor people, are oriented more often to the present than the future. This orientation, we have already seen, can have implications for how homeless people prioritize their health problems: conditions with immediate rather than future, consequences are going to attract their attention.

Provider Attitudes

Because many homeless persons are alienated from formal services and the medical profession, homeless health care providers should attempt to reengage their clients by proving they have something valuable to offer. To do this, providers should understand the homeless environment and adapt therapeutic strategies to this environment. In many cases, it will not be possible to address each of the patient's medical needs. As discussed earlier, providers, if they are to be effective in the long run, must first attend to the homeless person's perceived medical needs.

Experienced providers of care to the homeless have learned that regardless of their physical or psychological appearance, homeless individuals, like all of us, respond positively when they are treated with respect and dignity. Those with experience with this population have also learned that behavior, which at first seemed bizarre, made sense once viewed in the context of the everyday lives of their patients. Understanding the etiology of behaviors is not always sufficient to allow problems in service provision to be solved, but it does foster a tolerance and appreciation that goes a long way toward creating a more satisfying relationship between patient and provider.

CONCLUSION

In this chapter, we describe how the homeless environment, and the attitudes and beliefs of homeless individuals influence their decisions of whether to seek medical care, and their behavior once they do seek care. We also provide some suggestions of how health care can be structured to respond to the special needs of the homeless. Although health care workers cannot solve the complex problem of homelessness, they are in a unique position to ease the suffering of homeless people.

Case Management for Homeless Families: An Integrated Multidisciplinary Approach

3

Michael R. Cousineau, Mark Casanova, Robert Erlenbusch

CHAPTER HIGHLIGHTS

- Case management is critical in helping clients make their way through the highly specialized, bureaucratic, and fragmented system serving the homeless population.
- A variety of homeless providers (e.g., social workers, nurses, mental health workers, psychologists, and unlicensed community workers) can serve as case managers.
- Barriers to effective case management include bureaucratic obstacles in the social service network, sociocultural biases in the provider community, and clients' distrust of the health and social service system.
- Old cultural and economic stereotypes associated with homelessness may lead to an inappropriate approach to resolving clients' actual needs.
- A case management model has at its center the case manager who, working with other members of the health care team, coordinates the array of services needed by the homeless.
- The health care team should address the medical, psychosocial, environmental (housing), and survival (food, clothing, employment, and cash assistance) needs of clients.
- The practice of case management involves five major functions: intake (assessment and crisis intervention); goal setting; plan of

action (provision of services and referrals); follow-up; and advocacy and networking.
• Case managers should try to "put themselves out of work" by promoting political change to address the underlying causes of homelessness and poverty.

INTRODUCTION

The human service delivery system serving the homeless population is large and very complex. The system is also highly specialized, fragmented, and bureaucratic. System components, such as housing, health, cash assistance, child care, mental health, and food assistance, rarely coordinate services or even consult with each other on individual cases. Programs have different eligibility requirements and different application procedures. This fragmentation and lack of coordination results in access barriers for many homeless, particularly the most vulnerable populations of homeless, such as the mentally ill.

In this highly specialized and fragmented system, case management is critical. Homeless individuals and families find it extremely difficult to obtain social and health-related services in a timely fashion. A professional case manager can successfully link homeless people with needed resources. Good case management does more than simply provide information and referrals, however. It coordinates the services needed by homeless clients. Moreover, case managers are often able to establish a one-to-one relationship with clients and thus provide a form of counseling and therapy that promotes growth and self-sufficiency (Weil, 1985). Finally, case managers function at the community level to improve access to existing services as well as increase resources needed by homeless clients.

Case management is not the exclusive activity of any one professional group, although trained social workers (who receive a master of social work or licensed clinical social work degree) provide case management services in most agencies. Today, the term *case manager* is applied to many types of individuals including nurses, mental health workers, and psychologists. Further, in some agencies, unlicensed paraprofessional workers perform many case management functions, leaving counseling and therapy to licensed clinical psychologists and social workers (Rothman et al., 1988). Some models of case management create a multilevel system in which administrators, supervisors, social workers, and aides all have specialized functions ranging from macrolevel administration, networking, and system advocacy to microlevel work with clients (Austin & Caragonne, 1986; O'Connor, 1988).

Case management has been applied in work with many special populations including the physically and mentally disabled, people with AIDS, paroled felons, drug addicts, children displaced from families because of neglect or abuse, and senior citizens.

Increasingly, case management is being employed by agencies serving the homeless. Case management for the homeless population creates particular challenges to service providers because the homeless are often encountered in short-stay emergency shelters, day drop-in centers, and clinics where limited opportunities exist for comprehensive planning, follow-up, and case review. As a result, social services for the homeless are often limited to crisis intervention, information, and referral. Case management may be more effective for homeless individuals residing in transitional housing programs that allow 3- to 24-month stays.

BARRIERS TO EFFECTIVE CASE MANAGEMENT FOR THE HOMELESS

System Barriers

Case managers must be aware of the many barriers faced by homeless individuals and families seeking assistance. Most shelters, for example, do not have spanish-speaking staff, and are unwilling to accept people who use drugs or alcohol, or are disabled. Other shelters will not accept families, particularly families with older teenaged children. Few shelters are able to care for people with AIDS.

Homeless clients encounter other obstacles in their efforts to gain access to services and programs. Public assistance (welfare) offices where people must go for Aid to Families With Dependent Children (AFDC), General Assistance, Social Security, Medicaid or food-stamps, are generally inhospitable and highly bureaucratic. Long lines and extended waits in a crowded welfare office; a hostile and suspicious eligibility worker who is uninformed about current eligibility regulations, and a maze of forms and requirements that must be met are intimidating to many homeless, especially the mentally disabled.

The case manager can serve as an advocate for clients, instructing them about what to ask for, how to ask for it, who to ask, how to appeal if benefits are denied, and, if necessary, accompany them on their appointment. In one case, a case manager for a shelter accompanied a homeless woman and her child to the public assistance office after she was wrongly denied AFDC benefits. The case manager informed the eligibility worker that she had misinterpreted department eligibility regulations. After resolving the problem, the woman walked out of the office, not only with her first month's AFDC check, but also with food stamps and Medi-Cal (California's Medicaid program) for herself and her child.

Homeless people face similar obstacles in trying to gain access to health and human service programs. Like welfare offices, public health clinics, hospitals, alcohol detoxification and drug treatment programs, and mental health centers are often crowded, and the client faces long waits to see the health care or program workers. Financial screeners are often unavailable or uninformed about eligibility for assistance programs and may inappropriately charge clients fees before they get care.

Again, case managers can provide important advocacy and support services. They can make the appointment with the health facility, give the client a map and bus tokens, and provide the name of financial assistance programs for which the client is eligible. For example, in Los Angeles, the County's Department of Health Services has a sliding fee scale called "The Ability to Pay Plan" (ATP). Patients not on ATP are charged $25 to $35 for a clinic visit. Many eligibility workers either fail to inform patients about the ATP program or are uninformed about the county's own eligibility policies. In making referrals to county hospitals and clinics, case managers instruct their clients not to wait to be offered the program, but to ask for the ATP plan when they first walk in. They also instruct clients on how to respond if their request is denied. By providing this level of advocacy, case managers are empowering their clients to overcome the obstacles to self-sufficiency and independence.

Sociocultural Biases

Cultural and economic stereotypes associated with homelessness may lead to an inappropriate approach to resolving a client's actual problems. Common perceptions of the homeless as white middle-aged male alcoholics living on Skid Row, or as mentally ill, are no longer accurate. The homeless today are younger (middle to early 30s), increasingly black, increasingly female, and include many families.

To work with homeless people effectively, caregivers should first examine their assumptions about why people are homeless and their attitudes toward this population. Similarly, the case manager must recognize stereotypes, cultural biases, and other differences that might adversely affect decisions on who receives services or gains entrance into a program. A case manager may discriminate against those who act dangerous, smell bad, or are dirty, without considering the factors that account for the person's condition or behavior.

The longer one is homeless, the greater the loss of physical and mental health. Resocialization is as necessary as physical and mental rehabilitation. A homeless person's abusive or uncooperative behavior should be understood in the context of his or her immediate situation. Moreover, although addiction to drugs and alcohol, and mental illness continue to be found among many homeless people, transient drug use or situational (acute) depression may be misinterpreted as a more chronic, profound dysfunction, leading to an inappropriate referral or case management approach.

Client-Centered Barriers

The individual or family may exhibit certain personal emotional problems that prevent the case manager from establishing a therapeutic relationship with the client. Years of homelessness leave some people bitter. The homeless person may believe a case manager's assistance will deprive him or her of their freedom. Some homeless clients, albeit fewer than are generally perceived, are determined to be left alone and will reject any offers of assistance.

The homeless client may be apprehensive about working with the case manager because of prior negative experiences with the social service or health system. They also may not trust the network of caregivers referred by the case manager. This general distrust is sometimes reflected by showing up late or failing to appear for scheduled appointments, failing to comply with prescribed medication or other medical recommendations, or, as often happens, disappearing without making further contact. Working with mentally disabled clients may be particularly frustrating; even small successes often require many encounters during a long period during which the case manager builds trust and rapport with the client.

HEALTH CARE MODEL

Often, because of scarce resources and the barriers described earlier, services to the homeless are episodic and do little more than address the most pressing of client needs—a bed for the night, warm clothing, a meal, care for an acute medical condition. For interventions to have more lasting impact, they must be coordinated and persistent, addressing both the short-term and long-term needs of clients.

As in more traditional health care settings, such as hospitals and clinics, social workers play a key role in the case management process. With the homeless, however, we believe effective case management must actively involve other members of the health care team: nurses, physicians, mental health specialists, health educators, job counselors, and substance abuse specialists. Health care for the homeless could be viewed as case management. In this context, the health care team should address not just the medical, but the psychosocial, environmental (housing), and survival (food, clothing, employment, and cash assistance) needs of clients. This section describes such an effort—a model that, although meeting immediate needs, helps clients make fundamental change in their lives.

This model has, at its center, a case manager, who, working as part of a health care team, integrates the array of services needed by the homeless. The model is most appropriate for homeless clients living in transitional housing. Variations of the model are needed for clients living in less stable environments.

Social Worker

In health care settings, social workers remain at the center of the case management process. The social worker helps the individual confront the social and environmental problems that may have contributed to the person's homeless state: eviction, a chronic health problem, lack of adequate job training, or substance abuse. The social worker's job in helping to resolve the client's nonhealth care needs makes him or her an indispensable part of the health care team. In the role of case manager, the social worker participates in case review meetings with other health professionals and is available during clinical sessions for crisis intervention and consultation.

Health Care Practitioners

While the social worker is enrolling the family in Medicaid or cash assistance programs, obtaining housing vouchers or shelter, and food stamps or other social services, health care practitioners provide important health-related information and service to clients. Physicians and nurses prescribe an appropriate medical regimen (including medicines and ancillary care), and recommend appropriate referrals to other health care institutions. The nurse monitors medication, helps pregnant women obtain prenatal care, and ensures that children get immunized. The mental health specialist responds to psychological crises, identifies child abuse and other forms of domestic violence, and assesses mental illness and substance abuse. A health educator provides preventive education and health counseling including information about the spread of AIDS, nutrition, and ways to obtain food and other resources. Clearly, if the team is to work effectively, frequent multidisciplinary case conferences are necessary.

CASE MANAGEMENT FUNCTIONS

The practice of case management involves five major functions.

1. Intake: assessment and crisis intervention
2. Goal setting
3. Plan of action services and referral
4. Follow-up
5. System advocacy and networking

Although each function is discrete, increasingly case management involves the close linking and integration of these functions.

Intake: Assessment and Crisis Intervention

For most patients encountered during a health care visit or at a shelter, the case manager conducts an assessment of the primary or immediate needs of the client and his or her family. In addition to health problems, these needs may include emergency rent assistance, food, clothing, cash assistance including enrollment in public assistance programs, prenatal care for pregnant women and immunizations for children, residential detoxification if the client is chemically addicted, personal hygiene, employment, and secondary medical care.

Once the immediate crisis has subsided, and the family or individual placed in housing or shelter, the case manager can begin to address the clients' requirements for child care, employment, and outpatient or residential treatment for drug or alcohol dependence, and mental health. The case manager should learn as much about the history of the individual as possible. How long has the person or family been homeless? What led to the current homeless situation? Is the person or family enrolled in AFDC or Social Security Insurance, or do they receive food stamps or Medicaid? If not, are they eligible for these programs? Is he or she employed? Does the person have any job skills? Is there any evidence of mental illness, chronic illness, or substance abuse? Is there any evidence of domestic violence? The sample intake form (see Table 3.1) provides a structure for the intake assessment.

The case manager's first objective is to address the health conditions for which the patient is seeking assistance. Therefore, the case manager's role in most models will be limited to crisis intervention. The purpose of crisis intervention is to stabilize the individual or family. It is often the first step in case management of homeless individuals. Case managers must be prepared to assist the client find a shelter bed, a respite care bed, or a bed in a home for battered women and children. Case managers also provide psychosocial counseling and support, and intervene with public agencies to release rent assistance or public assistance checks. They should have at their disposal accurate up-to-date information about resources that can be obtained on short notice. Case managers should also get to know people in county or city social service departments who could be of assistance in resolving immediate crises. Because the need for shelter will be most immediate, case managers should understand the shelter system, particularly shelter locations, fees if any, restrictions, services offered, and number of beds. Crisis intervention also requires the case manager to understand other emergency support services. In California, for example, a federally sponsored emergency rent assistance program—FEMA (Federal Emergency and Management Assis-

Table 3.1 Sample Intake Form for Case Manager's Assessment of Homeless Persons' Needs

	Resources
Immediate crisis-oriented needs:	
Housing	HUD, Section 8, Red Cross Rental Assistance, Homeless Families Program (AB1733), board and care, shelters, transitional housing, independent living centers, food banks, WIC, Meals on Wheels, SNAP Program
Food	Department of Public Social Services, food pantries, churches, missions, drop-in
Financial assistance	SSI, DPSS (AFDC, GR), Employment Development Department, Veterans Administration Office, Medicaid/Medicare, Emergency After Hours Services (Sundowner)
Psychosocial counseling	Community mental health centers, Mental Health Association, county mental health centers, socialization programs, day treatment centers, hotlines (rape, suicide, domestic violence, child abuse, parenting classes, runaways, AIDS)
Health care	Free clinics, community clinics, dental clinics, country hospitals, county outpatient clinics, county health centers, Los Angeles County Medical Association
Drug and alcohol detoxification	County residential-outpatient treatment centers; community residential-outpatient treatment centers; substance abuse hotlines; AA, NA, ALANON, ACA groups
Medication monitoring and management	County mental health centers, psychiatric referral services, community mental health centers
Other (documents, clothing, advocacy)	Community social service agencies, information line, Legal Aid Foundation, Registrar-Recorder Office (vital statistics), Department of Motor Vehicles

38

Secondary needs:

Money management	Cost-free checking account, discount utility services (i.e., Lifeline)
Employment	EDD Office, private employment agencies, civil service agencies, *Yellow Pages*, chambers of commerce, business directories, newspaper advertisements
Child care	Child care information hotlines
Follow-up medical care	Free clinics, community clinics, dental clinics, county hospitals, county outpatient clinics, county health centers, Los Angeles County Medical Association
Ongoing mental health care	Community mental health centers, Mental Health Association, county mental health centers, socialization programs, day treatment centers, hotlines (rape, suicide, domestic violence, child abuse, parenting classes, runaways, AIDS, self-help groups)
Drug and alcohol rehabilitation	County residential-outpatient treatment centers; community residential-outpatient treatment centers; substance abuse hotlines; AA, NA, ALANON, ACA groups
Job training	Job Training Partnership Act Programs, Department of Rehabilitation, Public-private adult education schools, public-private occupational centers
Other follow-up (documents, clothing, advocacy)	Community social service agencies, information line, Legal Aid Foundation, Registrar-Recorder Office (vital statistics), Department of Motor Vehicles
Leisure-time resources	Public libraries, community parks and recreation centers, public zoos and museums, local YWCA and YMCA

tance,) run by the Red Cross, provides one month's rent to families able to show only minimal proof of homelessness.

Shelters and rent assistance programs enable case managers to find available housing quickly, even before other resources, such as Medicaid, welfare, or food stamps, are obtained.

Goal Setting

Once needs are assessed and the immediate crisis resolved, the case manager should establish a plan of action. Although a limited amount of goal setting occurs during crisis intervention, case managers must initially focus on stabilizing their clients and helping them make short-term commitments. Once the immediate crisis has subsided, the case manager shifts attention to the client's long-term needs. Goals are set that the client can reasonably achieve within a short period. Health practitioners must be part of any goal setting, particularly if they are helping the individual with an acute health crisis or working on the management and resolution of a chronic health problem.

Goal setting usually occurs a few days after assessment and crisis intervention. Clients might need a few days to "cool out," to think about the kinds of goals they want to achieve. The process of goal setting requires an attentive and understanding case management team that can assess the client's desire to change, his or her ability to do so, and accessible resources to help in this effort.

What an individual wants and what the case manager thinks the person needs may vary. The client may indicate that he or she wants an apartment, whereas the case manager may recognize the need for an alcohol recovery program, or a child's need for developmental screening, immunizations, and child care. Discussions between client and case manager lead to a negotiated set of goals that the client can both articulate and agree to. The client may not agree to all the goals the case manager wants and vice versa.

In addition to establishing goals, a homeless family or individual needs assistance in prioritizing how these goals will be met. The individual or family makes a decision about what is most likely to be accomplished in the short-term, and what can or should be put off until later.

Initial goals should be achievable. Commonly, a homeless individual or family has had a series of setbacks or failures. A few victories in achieving goals will increase confidence and help promote more long-lasting change. Finally, a time frame is set for completion of each goal.

To help meet certain goals, clients can be encouraged to attend groups held at shelters or at clinics that address specific needs. For example, the Los Angeles Homeless Health Care Project provides weekly parenting groups, informal rap groups, health issues groups, and groups on money management and household skills.

Plan of Action: Services and Referral

After initial goal setting, the case manager assists the client to obtain needed resources. This often involves setting up weekly group or individual counseling sessions and making effective referrals. On some occasions, the case manager can best serve homeless clients by accompanying them, as an advocate, to the referring agency. During such visits, the case manager helps clients apply for program benefits and makes sure that the agency worker complies with program regulations and requirements.

Effective Referrals

Several factors determine whether a referral will or will not be effective. First, the client must personally feel the need for and want the service offered by the referral agency. The client must be able to make an appointment with an agency, keep the appointment, and meet any requirement associated with the visit (e.g., bring required documents, telephone ahead to confirm appointment).

Often, clients do not follow up with appointments. Although this lack of follow-up can be frustrating to a case manager, he or she should remember that homeless persons have competing needs and other problems that may be blocking them from doing what they themselves want. Although the case manager may have a specific idea about what is most important for the client, the client may perceive other needs to be of higher priority. For example, a nurse at a health clinic once expressed frustration about a client who consistently failed to show up for his twice weekly tuberculosis medication. After she explained the importance of taking his medication, he continued to miss appointments. The nurse discovered that coming across town for his medication made it impossible for him to get a good place in line for dinner or a bed at a large downtown shelter. Getting his medication could mean sleeping on the street without anything to eat. For the client, a meal and a place to stay occupied a higher priority than did tuberculosis treatment.

A second important factor in making an effective referral is to ensure that the client has the necessary referral information. For example, before the client leaves the clinical setting, make sure he or she has the referral agency's correct telephone number and address, knows the exact time and place of the appointment, and has a list of documents needed for the appointment. Health care programs often use community maps showing where agencies are in relation to the clinic or shelter, and the buses or subways needed to travel to the agency (see chapter 4 on outreach by Smith). Checklists should be provided that outline the documents needed for applications to various entitlement programs (birth certificate, payroll check stubs, Medicaid stickers, immunization records for a child, etc.).

Finally, the case manager must be reasonably sure that the individual is being referred to an agency that is prepared to help him or her achieve a specific objective. We suggest setting up formal referral agreements with agencies, as well as informal linkages to individuals within referring agencies who can help your clients get needed resources. Before a client is sent to an agency, call ahead and give the contact person the name of the client being referred, the problem for which you are requesting assistance and the team's telephone number if there are any questions. We suggest handing the client a form indicating the name of the individual at the referral agency to be seen, why the person is being referred, and the name of the health care team case manager making the referral.

Case Review

At a minimum, case review is done with the individual or family on a weekly basis. Progress in goal achievement is reviewed, and goals are renegotiated with new approaches and time extensions when necessary. The case management team should also meet weekly to review cases and brainstorm on any problems or concerns of a particular case. Case review meetings are used to share ideas or new referral or resource possibilities.

Near the time of discharge from the program, the client and case manager should set new goals for the future. These will include arrangements for housing or other shelters, linkages to other support systems, and follow-up for health and mental health services.

Follow-Up

Ideally, follow-up is done after an individual or family leaves the program. Follow-up may involve an occasional home visit or telephone call by the case management team to see how the individual and family is doing, and if they have new setbacks, problems, or concerns.

Follow-up is very difficult and time-consuming because clients are so mobile. A new Los Angeles–based program attempting to provide comprehensive case management, including follow-up care to homeless families, is so overwhelmed with the demands of new clients seeking emergency housing that staff has little time to adequately follow up on clients already in their case load.

System Advocacy and Networking

Although case management helps homeless individuals and families, it does little to address the root causes of homelessness. More and better shelters, staffed by highly trained case managers, delivering more and better services to homeless people will not alone solve the crisis of homelessness. To address the systemic problem of homelessness, and to prevent the downward spiral of poor people into homelessness, we need a major shift in the political agenda and a massive infusion of funds for affordable housing, job training programs, accessible health and mental health care delivery systems, and a range of social service programs.

Case managers are in a unique position to be a catalyst for social and political change because they bridge the gap between the streets and the legislative chambers. By virtue of their familiarity with issues and problems of homeless people, case workers can play an important role in shaping public policy. Their day-to-day case advocacy provides a wealth of information and documentation grounded in the experiences of street people. In Los Angeles, for example, frontline workers have provided the backbone of testimony about the impact of health care cuts on the delivery of care to poor people. In 1988, the result of this kind of testimony helped to pressure the Board of Supervisors to restore more than $50 million in previously slated cuts. Again, in 1989, Los Angeles mental health workers staged several rallies and provided key testimony at a Board of Supervisors hearing to keep mental health care clinics open.

Frontline workers can also use their expertise to help ease bureaucratic barriers that keep homeless people from needed resources. One important step in this process is coalition building and networking. Case workers need a forum to share common, but separately held, "bits of reality." It is in these shared experiences that the larger picture of bureaucratic incompetence or interscience becomes clearer, and tactics and strategies to resolve these issues can be discussed. For example, in Los Angeles, a group of advocates for the homeless meet twice a month in what are called "welfare check-in" meetings (one meeting for those working with single adults and another for those working with families) to discuss current welfare regulations and issues that relate to the implementation of these regulations.

Not only can advocates speak in different forums for homeless people, but, of even greater importance, they can help poor and homeless people speak for themselves. For this to happen, the homeless need resources and technical assistance, such as office space, copying, telephones, computers, meals, and transportation. For example, in 1985, after the city of Los Angeles bulldozed down an encampment of homeless people called Justiceville, several organizations provided office space and other administrative support so that the homeless could continue their organizing effort.

Those who work in social services, then, are in an unusual position to go beyond individual case advocacy. The question arises, however, why should they? Why should case managers engage in systemic advocacy?

One very powerful reason is to avoid personal and professional burnout. Unfortunately, social service agencies often do not allow their frontline workers (e.g., case managers, intake workers, secretaries) to participate in conferences and coalition work or to provide testimony. This mistake could lead to a frustrated and emotionally spent staff. Staff who are providing direct service have difficult and demanding jobs, and can often feel overwhelmed at what seems an unending stream of people needing services. Providing time for the kinds of advocacy described here will remind the case worker that they work within a larger context, and that they can help change policies that affect their clients' well-being and their work. Case managers and other staff must feel that the daily Band Aids they place on homeless people are part of a larger solution. Providing crisis intervention, transportation, and other services should not be divorced from the larger issues of economic and social justice.

Finally, case managers must avoid the trap of institutionalizing their work. In focusing solely on improved assessment and referral skills, social service agencies run the real risk of becoming efficient bureaucracies for working with the poor. As agencies serving the homeless grow, and as directors become adept at program development and fund raising, they can lose the vision that links homeless programs to the larger systemic issues of homelessness. Ultimately, the challenge for case managers is to find ways to put themselves out of work by being a vehicle for political change that addresses the underlying causes of homelessness and poverty.

CONCLUSION

The complexity of the human service delivery system makes it very difficult for homeless people to obtain vital services. Case management provides a focal point for linking homeless people in need of health care to food, clothing, housing, public assistance, and job training programs. The transiency of homeless individuals and restrictions on length of stay at shelters reduce the ability of social workers to provide a comprehensive array of services that include follow-up. A case management model for health care workers is proposed to augment existing health care delivery programs serving the homeless. The model is a framework for those involved in case management to assess the immediate and long-term needs of clients, set goals, implement plans for resolving problems, and provide follow-up and advocacy. The model relies on the case management team consisting of the social worker at the center and health care practitioners, health educators, and mental health specialists. Advocacy for broad social change is suggested as a way to reduce staff burnout, and provide health care workers with an opportunity to bridge their work and experiences with efforts to address the broader social and economic causes of homelessness.

REFERENCES

Austin, D., Caragonne P. (1986). A comparative analysis of twenty-two settings using case management components. The Case Management Research Project. Austin: University of Texas at Austin, School of Social Work.

O'Connor, G. C. (1988). Case Management: Systems and practice. *The Journal for Contemporary Social Work,* 97–106.

Rothman, J. et al. (1988). *The practice of case management: A study of case managers' experiences and views.* Los Angeles: UCLA School of Social Welfare. Center for Child and Family Policy Studies.

Weil, M. (1985). *Case management in human service practice.* San Francisco: Jossey-Bass.

General Guidelines for Health Care Delivery to Homeless Adults and Families in Shelters and Outreach Sites

4

Mary H. Smith

CHAPTER HIGHLIGHTS

- Outreach health care teams take medical care to the homeless—to shelters, parks, detoxification centers, lunch and dinner lines, and other areas where the homeless live and congregate.
- Homeless health care projects have developed two forms of outreach health care delivery: (a) triage and screening clinics; and (b) outreach clinics.
- Triage and screening clinics are located in alleys, beaches, lunch lines, and other community sites, providing nurse assessment and triage services.
- Outreach clinics provide a more comprehensive range of services in drop-in centers including partial or complete physical examinations, health and mental health services, and education.
- A triage and screening clinic is staffed by a midlevel practitioner or nurse and a clinic coordinator; an outreach clinic is usually staffed by a larger multidisciplinary team providing health, social, educational, and psychiatric services.
- The outreach health team should develop the knowledge and resources to make referrals for homeless clients to appropriate community resources for food, clothing, housing, income entitlements, advocate assistance, and additional community health clinic or hospital services.

- Outreach teams should carefully investigate all referral sources and follow-up on all referrals to ensure services were obtained.
- Supplies and medications needed for outreach care depend on the the personnel available, physical constraints of outreach sites, and the comprehensiveness of services.
- In addition to providing early identification of acute and chronic disease, outreach teams serve as patient advocates and educate both shelter guests and staff on preventive health measures.

INTRODUCTION

Outreach health care services are defined as the provision of health services by a trained professional medical team to a homeless population residing in shelters, parks, detoxification centers, or any other area where homeless people live or congregate.

Outreach health care services provide homeless adults and families with a unique opportunity to obtain access to primary care. The traditional medical model, in which the client comes to the outpatient clinic or hospital emergency department, often poses a formidable barrier for the homeless in need of medical care. The outreach clinic, by taking health care to the homeless in their own environment, removes this barrier.

The concept of outreach health care delivery finds its roots in the public health nursing model of home visits to individuals and family groups in the community. This model has been in existence for decades and is the mainstay of community-public health. Health promotion, disease identification, case finding, referrals for treatment, and patient and community education are an integral part of community-public health nursing. The outreach health care team performs the preceding activities but, in addition, has clinical expertise to diagnose and manage specific health problems in the field.

There are several advantages in taking health care to homeless people including early identification and treatment of acute and chronic disease, opportunity to promote better treatment compliance, and reinforcement of the need for follow-up care or visits. Meeting people in their own living situation, whether on the streets or in lunch lines, communicates to them a willingness to meet their health needs regardless of the setting.

This chapter provides information on the structure and function of outreach clinic teams. The specific areas to be discussed include outreach site staffing and structure; required medications and other supplies; the role of the outreach team in disease prevention, early disease identification and detection of comprehensive health problems; and the role of the outreach clinic team in client education and advocacy.

STAFFING AND STRUCTURE OF OUTREACH SITE

Two different forms of outreach health care delivery have been successfully implemented in the Homeless Health Care Projects across the United States: (a) triage and screening clinics; and (b) outreach clinics.

Triage and Screening Clinics

Triage and screening clinics are located in alleys, beaches, lines, and other community sites that do not have a room or privately screened-off area for a complete physical examination. A triage clinic is staffed by a midlevel practitioner or nurse and a clinic coordinator. The nurse or midlevel practitioner assesses and evaluates clients presenting with acute or chronic physical or mental health problems, and makes appropiate referrals. The clinic coordinator helps establish outreach sites, maintains the equipment, stocks supplies, helps set up the clinic, implements referrals, maintains patient records, pursues medical and social service referrals, and checks up on no-show patients.

The outreach model employs a proactive approach to client contact. Health team members approach individual clients; introduce themselves; and inquire about physical, mental, or social service problems the homeless individual may be experiencing. A personal, sensitive, and nonthreatening approach is always maintained. This approach often elicits specific health needs and problems the client was not even aware of, or had forgotten (e.g., dental pain or repair of broken glasses). Concrete and useful written information about community resources is then given to the homeless client. (See Community Referral Sheet).

Although triage and screening are critical components of the health care system for the homeless, they alone are not sufficient to meet the overall health needs of homeless individuals. It is a disservice to identify health problems if the outreach team is then unable to provide specific referrals to an outpatient clinic or social service agency. Triage and screening must always be viewed as a part of a comprehensive health care service delivery system.

Outreach Clinics

The second form of outreach health care delivery is full clinic services located at homeless drop-in centers or shelters. Outreach clinics integrate triage and screening with a more comprehensive health examination.

The goals of outreach clinics include early identification, diagnosis, management, and follow-up of health problems; disease prevention; health education; patient advocacy; and ongoing shelter staff education.

The staffing of outreach clinics should ideally consist of a nurse practitioner and physician, clinic coordinator, clinic assistant(s), nurses, social worker, therapist, and health educator(s). Any combination of the preceding staffing is feasible. Often, the core staff consists of a nurse practitioner and clinic coordinator. Factors that will determine the staffing and structure of outreach clinics include the composition and size of the homelesss population at the center or shelter, room availability, privacy, shelter staff cooperation, and the types of illnesses encountered.

The nurse practitioner and physician are primarily responsible for the evaluation, examination, and ongoing management of the overall health of the homeless person. The clinician, in collaboration with the clinic coordinator, social worker or therapist, and the patient, assesses the physical, psychological, and social service strengths and weaknesses of each individual. As with triage and screening clinics, the clinic coordinator is responsible for patient follow-up. The coordinator's tasks include assisting with the dispensing of medications, filling out requests and making referrals for laboratory examinations or radiographs, providing mental health or social service referrals, offering patient education, ensuring appropiate follow-up care, and supervising the clinic assistants.

The clinic assistants are responsible for creating the medical record, taking vital signs, assisting with patient flow, helping to provide patient education, and assisting with environmental safety and comfort.

At a mimimum, the outreach clinic should be held in a screened-off area in the corner of a room where examinations can be performed in a semiprivate setting. The optimum examination area is a separate room that can be locked to ensure quiet and privacy. The room should include an examination table with stirrups for gynecological examinations. Completing patient registration and taking vital signs should occur away from the examining area and crowded areas of the shelter to provide the patient with privacy and confidentiality. Only patients or family members of patients to be examined should be allowed in the clinic area.

An outreach clinic at the largest family shelter in Los Angeles demonstrates how outreach health services are implemented. The outreach team had several meetings with the shelter staff to document the specific health care needs and concerns of the shelter residents and staff. The shelter staff designated that the dining hall and an office located in the basement of the church be used as examination areas. The office serves as a private examination room, and the dining hall is partitioned off with portable partitions, creating three separate semiprivate examination areas. Dining room tables, set up in the basement, are used to complete patient registration, to take vital signs, and to dispense medications. A separate waiting area for patients is set up at the far end of the dining room, away from the examination areas. Another dining table near the waiting area is used for patient education. Children whose parents or siblings are waiting to be evaluated are entertained by volunteers with health-oriented art projects. The children learn a great deal and have fun while the parents or adults are freed up to see the practitioner.

In a separate location from the dining hall, the clinic coordinator and a clinic assistant perform triage of health problems of clients' waiting to be seen. Then they create a medical outreach record. After registering, the clinic assistant brings residents to the dining room where the intake and examination are completed. Following the examination, residents wait in the designated area for medications, counseling, referrals, and follow-up appointments.

Because of the lack of privacy, only partial physical examinations can be performed at the shelter. Patients requiring a more extensive physical examination are referred back to the base community clinic. The outreach team is able to provide several mental health interventions including counseling for depression, anxiety, and situational stress; social service information on entitlements and substance abuse programs; and ongoing case management.

The team provides health and mental health services to the shelter once a week, seeing between 10 to 15 patients. The setup, implementation, and cleanup for this particular off-site clinic is completed in a 3-hour period.

The staff nurse pratitioner and clinic coordinator follow up and review each outreach medical record the morning following each site visit. The nurse practitioner then calls the public health nurse assigned to the shelter to alert him or her to potential communicable disease cases, child abuse or neglect cases, and any information pertinent to the overall health of the shelter residents and staff.

An outreach clinic at the shelter allows the shelter staff to become involved with the health needs of residents and to help identify residents that are in need of health services. The outreach clinic often provides medical and mental health services that the residents have needed for months but have not received. A mother may sign her infant up to be examined for a cold and at the same time inquire about family planning services for herself; an elderly woman with sores on her feet and arms may be diagnosed with diabetes; a young man, feeling suicidal and depressed, can obtain immediate psychiatric intervention.

REFERRAL

The triage and screening team and outreach clinics will encounter many health and social problems that are beyond their scope of intervention. To be effective, they must refer clients to appropiate community resources for food, clothing, housing, income entitlements, advocate assistance, and community clinics or hospital services. The information given to homeless clients should be tested by the health team for accuracy, and the referral agency should be tested for access barriers. The health team also should meet regularly with local agencies to discuss unsuccessful referrals and how to improve interagency referrals.

Common barriers that keep the homeless from obtaining services are: (a) lack of communication between the agencies regarding the specific need of the homeless person, (b) lack of knowledge of what services a particular agency can or cannot provide, (c) lack of transportation, and (d) unrealistic appointment times. Any referral problems identified by the team or homeless clients need to be addressed on an ongoing basis. Generally, when establishing referral sources, clinics should do the following:

- Meet with the referral agency staff to tour the facility and obtain an overview of services offered, hours open, and service limitations; and exchange information about the clinic's facility with the referral staff.

- Identify a specific contact(s) person at the agency who can be called when a problem arises.
- Establish how the referrals should be made (e.g., referral note, telephone call).
- Follow up with telephone calls to the agency after sending a client, if referral or communication problems occur.

The following is an example of how a local drop-in center facilitated the referral of a mentally confused and wheelchair-bound patient to our community clinic. The center called ahead and alerted the clinic staff to the specific health problems of the individual, arranged transportation to and from the clinic, and sent a referral note with the patient. The referral went smoothly, and the clinic was able to provide appropriate care to the individual.

In general, the clinic coordinator follows up on referral problems. She or he identifies the problem, contacts the referral agency, and works with the agency staff on ways to complete the referral. The coordinator regularly reports back to the team and individual client on the range of available referrals, procedures to be followed, and referral contact persons.

It is essential for the outreach team to develop a referral sheet that describes available food, shelter, and health and mental health services specific to the health team's service catchment area. The referral sheet provides a map of the service area with specific written information about the referral agencies, and their addresses, services, hours, and contact persons. Often, the referral sheet acts as a compass in orienting the newly arrived homeless person to street names, bus lines, and directions.

SUPPLIES AND MEDICATIONS

The types of supplies and medications the health team uses at the outreach clinic site will be determined by the specific health problems found; type of physical examination possible; and the range of laboratory, radiological, and diagnostic tests available at the base clinic or in the community. The Homeless Outreach Team at the Venice Family Clinic has established seven outreach clinics in the community. At all sites, the lack of a private examination room permits only the examinations of patients from the waist up. Patients needing pelvic or genital examinations, or more complete diagnostic examinations (e.g., electrocardiogram [EKG], audiometry) are seen at the base community clinic the same or following day.

Tables 4.1 and 4.2 contain suggestions for supplies and medications used in an outreach clinic setting. Supplies and over-the-counter medications can be stored and transported in lightweight plastic tubs with handles. Prescription drugs and immunizations requiring refrigeration can be stored and transported in a Playmate cooler with ice packs. Clinic forms, medical records, health education materials, and miscellaneous forms can be carried in a bin with handles. Depending on the site, the health team may store the supplies and medications in a locked area at the outreach site, or transport them between the outreach site and the community-based clinic.

Table 4.1 Supplies Used in Outreach Clinic

Ace bandages
Alcohol wipes
Band-aids
Betadine solution
Bili-lab stix
Stool cans for enteric cultures
Contaminated waste box
Cotton balls
Culturettes
Ear specula
Regular, extra-large, and child blood pressure cuffs
First-aid kit
Flashlight
Foam pad—6' long, 2' wide
Funnel
Gloves
Hemoglobinometer
Kidney basin
Kleenex
Lubricating jelly
WIC (Women, Infants, Children) appointment referrals
Bus tokens
Clinic forms
Directions, maps
Health education materials
Immunization consents

Moisturizing lotion
Ophthalmoscope
Otoscope
Paper bags
Paper cups
Paper drapes
Paper towels
Pill bottles and vials with prescription labels
Pill counter set
Q-tips
Rantex wipes
Sterilized urine containers
Stethoscopes
Sunscreen
Syringes (3ml, 5ml)
Syringes and needles (for tuberculosis and immunizations)
Tape
Tape measure
Tongue depressors
Triangular bandage
4×4 gauze
Pens, paper clips
Records of patient progress notes
Prescription pads
Referral notebooks

Table 4.2 Medications Used in an Outreach Clinic

Analgesics and Anti-inflammatories
Aspirin, (325 mg tablets)
Motrin, (400 mg tablets)
Tylenol; drops, elixir, (325-mg tablets)
Antiobiotics:
Amoxicillin elixir (125 mg, 250 mg/ 5 ml
Ampicillin (250-mg, 500-mg (tablets)
Bactrim DS tablets
Bactrim suspension
Dicloxacillin 250 mg tabs, elixir 62.5 mg/ 5ml
Enthromycin oral suspension 200 mg/ 5ml
Enthromycin; (250-mg tablets)
Nystatin oral suspension
Penicillin VK (250-mg tablets, elixir, 250 mg/5 ml)
Tetracycline (250-mg tablets)
Cold Medicines:
Actifed tablets
Antihistamine and cold remedy syrups
Chlortrimetron (4 mg tablets)
Sudafed (60 mg tablets)
Creams and Ointments:
Bacitracin ointment
Hydrocortisone cream (0.5% and 1%)
Lotrimin Cream, Nystatin ointment and cream
Triamcinolone cream (0.025% and 0.1%)

Miscellaneous:
Alupent spray
Alupent syrup
Antacids
Atarax (25-mg tablets)
Benadryl (5-mg and 50-mg tablets, syrup, (12.5 mg/5 ml)
Beclovent oral spray
Cortisporin otic suspension
Immunizations, syringes (tuberculosis: 3 ml, 5 ml)
Iron (220-mg tablets), elixir, drops
Kwell lotion and shampoo with combs
Nifedipine (20 mg-tablets)
Pedalyte
Sulfacetamide (ophthalmologic solution)
Theophylline (50-, 100-, 300-mg tablets)
Vasocon-A (ophthalmologic solution)

EARLY IDENTIFICATION AND MANAGEMENT OF HEALTH PROBLEMS

The primary concern of the health care team is identification and proper management of acute and chronic health problems. Acute

health problems commonly seen in outreach clinics include incomplete or lost immunization records, ear infections, upper-respiratory infections, asthma, bronchitis, pneumonia, impetigo, cellulitis,
lacerations, trauma, fungal infections, infestations of lice and scabies, gastroenteritis, and sexually transmitted diseases. Mental health
problems commonly encountered are altered mental status, suicidal
ideation, substance abuse, schizophrenia, depression, anxiety, dual
diagnosis, family violence, child abuse, and family dysfunction.

Chronic health problems often seen in homeless adults include
hypertension, diabetes, thyroid dysfunction, heart disease, chronic
obstructive pulmonary disease, arthritis, peripheral vascular disease,
AIDS risk factors, AIDS, substance abuse, depression, schizophrenia,
and anxiety. In children, common chronic health problems include
physical growth delay, failure to thrive, chronic otitis media, developmental delays, asthma, eczema, behavioral problems, and depression. Often, parents have failed to obtain follow-up for previously
diagnosed, long-standing health problems.

An outreach team consisting of a midlevel clinician and clinic
coordinator can evaluate most of these physical and mental health
problems, and implement an initial treatment plan. Complex medical or psychological problems should be more thoroughly evaluated
and managed by a team composed of a physician, midlevel clinician,
nurse, social worker, and clinic coordinator either at the outreach
site or the community-based clinic.

DISEASE PREVENTION

Through early identification and management of acute and
chronic health problems, the health care team can initiate primary
and secondary prevention of disease. The outreach team should perform ongoing survelliance of the health and safety of shelters or
drop-in sites. They should institute measures to prevent the transmission of communicable diseases, accidents, injuries, child abuse and
neglect, and mental illness.

The prevention of communicable disease outbreaks by shelter personnel requires daily cleaning and maintenance of bathrooms, sleeping areas, and food preparation areas. The transmission of disease via
the fecal–oral route can be prevented by the proper disposal of diapers in a designated trash can, use of diaper changing tables, and

good hand washing. Food handlers must be routinely screened for potential health problems such as infectious diarrhea, hepatitis, or tuberculosis.

The prevention of accidents and injuries in a sheltered population requires that the shelter install safety gates at stairwells, create a supervised play area, child-proof the living and play area in the shelter or center, and encourage shelter staff to provide surveillance and maintenance of environmental safety.

Prevention of potential child abuse and neglect can be assisted by on-site parenting classes; early identification of parent(s) who may be at risk for, or have a past history of, abuse; and on-site counseling services for crisis intervention and family case management. The health care team, in cooperation with shelter or drop-in staff and the public health nurse, must constantly assess the parenting abilities of homeless families and provide comprehensive support before child abuse and neglect occur.

Primary prevention of mental illness requires accessible mental health services, and the development of a personal and trusting relationship between the health team and the clients they serve. The development of new situational anxiety, insomnia, or hypochon-driacal symptoms may be the first signs of stress caused by homeless-ness. The shelter and health care personnel should be encouraged to offer a homeless person an opportunity to cry, express anger, or seek guidance in the often chaotic atmosphere of the shelter. Often, the personal relationship between an outreach team member and a patient enables the patient to feel comfortable enough to see a psychi-atrist, go to parenting classes, or take a psychotropic medication. Mental health intervention is emotionally taxing and time-consum-ing. Nevertheless, it is critical. The health care team can often effec-tively intervene to get help for mentally troubled homeless clients.

PATIENT-CLIENT EDUCATION AND ADVOCACY

Patient education is another important responsibility of all out-reach clinics. Patient education should include self-care skills such as wound care, temperature taking, hand washing, teeth brushing, proper disposal of dirty diapers, and following safety measures in the home and car. Our outreach clinic at a local family shelter enlists the services of trained volunteer health educators to discuss and teach basic self-care skills to families. Use of audiovisual aids such as coloring books, thermometers, and puppets allows the families to learn by participation and have fun at the same time. Demonstrations that review basic hygiene and disease prevention should be kept simple to foster greater attention and participation of shelter guests.

The health team is consistently providing information regarding health maintenance issues such as substance abuse prevention and education, the need for annual Papanicolaou (Pap) and Mantoux tests and hemoculture testing in adults older than 40 years of age, birth control, immunizations (adults and children), yearly physicals, and assessment of risk factors for AIDS exposure.

As part of the educational effort, health care teams act as patient advocates. Advocacy is defined as pleading or defending the cause of another through information or direct action. Health care delivery to a homeless population or, for that matter, any population would not be complete without such advocacy. The outreach team serves as an advocate by providing information to the client on community resources for food, housing, clothing, case management, entitlements, and health, mental health, and substance abuse programs.

SHELTER STAFF EDUCATION

The final goal of the outreach team is to educate the staff at the shelter or drop-in site on issues related to the physical and mental health needs of clients and staff. Shelter or drop-in site staff needs information and training on environmental safety and hygiene, child abuse, substance abuse and treatment, ways to screen for common acute and chronic health conditions, and common mental health symptoms and behaviors.

The outreach team should emphasize the shelter staff's need for routine cleaning of bathrooms and common eating and sleeping areas, proper storage of perishable food and milk, disposal of trash (particularly soiled diapers), proper storage of medications, vector and vermin control, and maintenance of a complete first-aid kit.

Education about child abuse identification and reporting is also of critical importance. Staff members should know that they are mandated to report suspected cases of child abuse or neglect as well as reporting cases that have clear evidence of child abuse or neglect. In coordination with the health department and child protective services, the outreach team should educate shelter or site staff on the proper reporting and follow-up procedures for child abuse. More important, teaching staff the skills of prevention and early identification of high-risk parents could prevent future abuse by other parents.

Finally, the outreach team should teach the shelter staff the physical manifestations and behavioral changes that occur with drug or alcohol addiction, and procedures for making referrals to local drug and alcohol programs. Parental drug or alcohol abuse often is associated with child abuse or neglect. The shelter staff should know how to assess parents for both substance abuse and the quality of their parenting skills before child abuse or neglect occurs. Parents with alcohol or drug abuse problems need an urgent referral to a drug or alcohol treatment program, and continued surveillance for parental competency.

As with physical health problems, drug or alcohol abuse should be assessed and managed in a direct manner. Shelter staff need specific guidelines for handling clients under the influence of drugs or alcohol. We have used role playing and sharing of specific case examples to illustrate and teach shelter staff how to manage a person under the influence of a drug.

The Venice Family Clinic outreach staff, the county's public health nurse, and shelter staff meet quarterly, and more often if needed, to help the site staff identify problems and make appropiate referrals. We believe our efforts have enhanced services to the clients and have helped build the staff's confidence with regard to their assessment skills.

Inservice training seminars enable the shelter or drop-in center staff to assist the health care team in recognizing health care problems early, and to institute proper management and treatment. Seminar topics include basic first aid, cardiopulmonary resuscitation training, burnout, confidentiality, privacy, case conferencing and networking with other agencies, triage for routine and emergency health problems, screening for communicable diseases, common acute and chronic health prob ems, identification and implementation of appropiate referrals for mental illness, and identification and reporting of child abuse and neglect.

CONCLUSION

Health care delivery to homeless adults and families in shelters and outreach sites can be implemented effectively using an interdisciplinary team approach. Knowledge of client populations, early identification of acute and chronic diseases, disease prevention, patient education, advocacy, and shelter staff education are all important components in providing comprehensive care to a disenfranchised population. Working together, the health care team and the shelter staff can effectively provide medical and emotional support to the homeless population.

Preventive Medical Care for Homeless Men and Woman

5

Linda Weinreb

CHAPTER HIGHLIGHTS

- Homeless adults are at high risk for a variety of illnesses that can either be prevented, or detected and effectively treated in their early stages.
- Because of their acute care needs, preventive services for the homeless are too often overlooked.
- Homeless patients usually seek care for acute medical problems; visits for acute problems should be used to provide preventive care services.
- Providers should develop a simple preventive health plan based on the age, gender, individual risk factors, and common conditions of the homeless population they serve.
- All homeless adults should receive immunizations to prevent diptheria, tetanus, influenza, pneumococcal pneumonia and hepatitis.
- All homeless adults should be offered BP screening; yearly TB skin testing; routine cultures or serologies for sexuality transmitted diseases, including AIDS; breast, cervical , and colon examinations; yearly cholesterol-level testing; and tonometry screening for glaucoma.
- Homeless health care providers should provide birth control counseling to homeless women of child-bearing age during all

visits, even when the visit is for unrelated problems. Each birth
control method presents its unique problems for homeless women
and should be thoroughly discussed.

INTRODUCTION

Homeless adults are a heterogeneous group whose members require a wide range of preventive and routine health services. The
nature of these services is, in most ways, the same as in the general
adult population: screening measures, early identification and treatment of medical problems, and education to promote a healthy life-
style and minimize behaviors that pose the risk of adverse health
outcomes.

Although preventive services required by homeless adults are similar to that provided to a non-homeless population, providing these
services is often more challenging for practitioners. Disease prevention services may seem almost ludicrous in the acute or chronic crisis
of homelessness. Nevertheless, homelessness is most often a transient
condition, and the health care team must treat not only acute health
needs but promote long term health. Furthermore, although resolving homelessness is the most important preventive health intervention, other health prevention activities can make a significant difference in the well-being of homeless persons.

Homeless adults are at high risk for a variety of illnesses, such as
cancer, hypertension, tuberculosis, and dental disease, that can
either be prevented or detected and effectively treated in their early
stages. Conditions associated with homelessness also complicate preventive care. Poor nutrition, for example, can greatly compromise
individuals with hypertension or diabetes. Moreover, the stress of
homelessness financial barriers, and a complex, fragmented health
care system make it difficult to obtain care, especially preventive
medical care. This chapter reviews health promotion and preventive
services for homeless adults. In addition, general guidelines and
recommendations for health evaluations and a preventive health
plan for this population is presented.

PREVENTIVE HEALTH MEASURES

Although some controversy exists about the content, frequency,
and effectiveness of various preventive health measures, the im-

portance of preventive medical care for adults is unquestioned. It is helpful to think about preventive health care and routine medical care for homeless adults in two broad categories: (a) health promotion and protection; and (b) preventive medical services.

Health Promotion and Protection

Health promotion consists primarily of educational and intervention services that encourage healthy behavior including nutrition counseling, AIDS education and counseling, alcohol and drug abuse education, and smoking cessation strategies. Health personnel based in clinics or those doing outreach can provide health education and counseling to clients during one-on-one sessions or during special group sessions. For example, in Worcester, Massachusetts, the physician who supervises local health services for homeless adults conducts a weekly smoking cessation group at the largest city's adult shelter. In some communities, volunteers with health backgrounds conduct health education sessions for homeless persons. Medical students or hospital-based residents on outreach teams can also help. For example, family practice residents in a Worcester training program are required to conduct several health education sessions at local shelters during their community medicine rotation. Shelter workers, trained by health staff in relevant health promotion areas such as nutrition and AIDS education can also provide homeless adults with basic health education.

When time allows, health promotion education and related referrals should be incorporated into clinic visits for acute health problems. Because of limited time and resources, it is particularly important to target those individuals at highest risk. For example, the provision of nutrition counseling, substance abuse, and AIDS education is critical for all homeless pregnant women. Likewise, practitioners should make the provision of AIDS counseling for intravenous drug users a priority. Clinic staff who should be available to provide health promotion education to clients include health workers, nurses, midlevel practitioners, and physicians.

Health protection aims to preserve the health and well-being of individuals. Health protection services that are especially important for homeless adults include the provision of adequate and safe shelter, the surveillance and control of infectious diseases at shelters, and the provision of preventive and restorative dental care.

Measures to secure temporary shelter, and eventually permanent housing, for homeless adults should be a goal of all health care intervention. As discussed in Chapter 4 by Smith, social workers or case managers working in outreach teams should take responsibility for helping individuals find housing.

Homeless health care providers are also responsible for screening and control measures for common infectious diseases. Often, health practitioners working with local health departments develop strategies to screen homeless adults for tuberculosis and facilitate appropriate follow-up (see chapter 12 by Panosian on tuberculosis). A substantial and cooperative effort is generally required among providers to screen individuals, check results, and track those persons who require further evaluation and medication. For example, in a program in Boston, one nurse is assigned solely to coordinate this effort.

The lack of preventive and restorative dental services are frequently a significant problem for homeless adults. Most communities have few dentists who accept Medicaid or are willing to see homeless persons. Dental services for homeless adults are often limited to emergency dental care (e.g., extractions) at publicly funded hospitals.

Despite these difficult realities, providing homeless persons with dental services is essential. Although services will vary in availability and extent depending on local resources, several options exist. These include either referring clients to local dental schools for care, or providing preventive and restorative dental care at shelter sites using volunteer dentists or dental students.

Development of institutional backup from dental schools, local dental facilities, and dentists is needed for more extensive dental care (e.g., restorative work, dentures, etc.) In a program in Boston, for example, a dentist and hygienist perform preventive and restorative care at shelter sites. Homeless patients are referred to two dental schools for more serious dental needs.

Preventive Medical Services

Preventive medical services aim to prevent medical problems, to detect diseases before they cause symptoms, and to identify and treat medical conditions early. For homeless adults, these services include physical examinations; immunizations; family planning and prenatal care; and screening for acute, chronic, and infectious diseases and tuberculosis. Many health organizations have developed recommendations for preventive health measures (American Cancer Society, 1980; Canadian Task Force, 1984). A complete discussion of preventive care recommendations is beyond the scope of this chapter. Several preventive interventions that are particularly important for the homeless adult population are discussed subsequently, however.

Periodic Examinations

Ideally, all adults should be scheduled for periodic health examinations and should receive all of the recommended screening measures. Unfortunately, the special circumstance of homelessness makes this ideal impossible to reach. In general, a homeless patient's visits for acute medical problems offer the best chance to provide preventive care. When presented with a complicated or difficult homeless patient, or when the practitioner is pressed for time, preventive measures can be targeted to the age, sex, and specific conditions for which homeless adults are at high risk. When there are fewer constraints, comprehensive health promotion, protection, and preventive services should be reviewed with the homeless client. Some of this information can be provided during the physical examination. For example, the practitioner can discuss the adverse effects of smoking while examining a client for a sore throat. The importance of providing age- and sex-appropriate preventive health care during acute care visits should be stressed when training and supervising new providers. In some instances, volunteers or auxiliary personnel can be trained to cover these topics.

Immunizations

Diphtheria tetanus, the only immunization indicated for all adults, is commonly overlooked in both the general and adult populations. If an individual has received a full primary tetanus series, they require boosters at 10-year intervals. Often, the homeless adult may not remember when he last had a tetanus booster. Unless there are specific contraindications, homeless adults without a clear history of a tetanus booster should be immunized.

Rubella vaccination should be offered to homeless women of childbearing age who are not pregnant and who are antibody negative, and who have no other contraindications for vaccination. When the practitioner is unable to perform serological testing, the woman should be questioned about whether or not she recalls having had a rubella vaccination. If there is no clear history of past rubella vaccination and if pregnancy is denied, the practitioner should vaccinate the patient. Newly vaccinated women should be advised to avoid pregnancy for 3 months. They should also be advised of the risk of congenital rubella syndrome if pregnancy occurs within 3 months of vaccination. This risk is theoretical, however, and should not preclude vaccination of potentially susceptible women.

Influenza vaccination is indicated annually in the fall for all homeless persons aged 65 or older, and persons suffering from asthma, chronic cardiopulmonary disorders, metabolic diseases (e.g., diabetes), immunosuppression, or renal failure.

Pneumovax should be administered to homeless individuals with increased susceptibility to pneumococcal pneumonia including the elderly, alcoholics, and persons with medical conditions (e.g., chronic cardiac or pulmonary disease, asplenia, diabetes, immunosuppression, etc.) that increase their risk of infection.

Homeless adults are at high risk for hepatitis B, and administration of hepatitis B vaccine should be considered, especially for intravenous drug users, homosexual men, and the sexual partners of these groups. Three doses of vaccine are given at time zero, and at 1 and 6 months. Patients should be given an immunization card and followed up aggressively. This will greatly increase the chances of completing the immunization series. Hepatitis B vaccine can often be obtained free from local health departments.

Screening Measures

Certain screening procedures should be offered to all homeless adults at their first visit to the clinic. Outreach clinics and health promotion teams can also perform some of these measures. Blood pressure screening should be a routine component of patient evaluation regardless of presenting problem. Blood pressure screening, which is generally nonthreatening, can also be offered at shelter sites and soup kitchens. Hypertension is very common among the homeless and leads to increased risk of cardiovascular and cerebrovascular morbidity and mortality (see chapter 6 by Fleishman and Farnham on chronic disease). Benefits of adequate antihypertensive therapy are clear. When possible, a diagnosis of hypertension should be based on multiple blood pressure determinations.

Tuberculosis screening should be performed yearly for all homeless adults because they are an extremely high-risk group (see chapter 12 by Panosian on tuberculosis). Adults without a clear history of past testing should be screened. Because the tuberculin test must be read at 48 hours, tuberculin screening can often be performed more effectively at outreach sites where follow-up is more likely.

Effective tuberculin testing requires a cooperative effort among the local public health department, outreach nurses, and shelter staff. In many communities, one individual (often a nurse) is responsible for tuberculin screening and follow-up. Networks must be developed with shelters, clinics, drop-in centers, and other places where the homeless congregate to facilitate screening, follow-up, and medication administration. In Boston, for example, the Pine Street Adult Shelter has an X-ray machine on site to perform chest radiographic screening for all adults with a positive PPD (purified protein derivative) test.

Screening for *sexually transmitted diseases* (STDs) is also of critical importance. Individuals at risk for STDs (syphilis, gonorrhea, chlamydia) include persons who engage in sex with multiple partners, prostitutes, and those who have a sexual partner with an STD. The prevalence of STDs observed among homeless adults is approximately equal to that of the general population (Wright & Weber, 1987). STDs are commoner among homeless women than men at all ages. As would be expected, however, the rate of STDs is greatest in individuals younger than 30 years of age and drops significantly in persons older than 50 years of age.

Sexually active homeless women should be screened yearly for chlamydia and gonorrhea. This can be done during a routine visit or included in visits for unrelated problems. Sexually active homeless men and women should also be periodically screened for syphilis. The optimal frequency of such screening, however, has not been established and should be left to the clinical discretion of the practitioner. All pregnant women and individuals who describe a recent exposure to an STD should receive these screening tests.

Homeless adults at risk for human immunodeficiency virus (HIV) infection include intravenous drugs users, homosexual men, and women whose past or present partners were HIV positive, intravenous drugs users, or bisexual. In addition to providing AIDS education and information on high-risk behaviors and prevention strategies to all homeless individuals, people who fall into these groups should be offered HIV testing (see chapter 8 by Avery and O'Connell on AIDS).

Cancer Screening

A breast examination should be performed yearly for all homeless women. A baseline mammogram is recommended for women between the ages of 35 to 40. During years 40 to 50, screening mammograms are indicated at one- or two-year intervals. Homeless women who are 50 years of age or older should receive yearly mammograms.

Many homeless women are at high risk for cervical cancer because of the presence of several risk factors such as low socioeconomic status, multiple sexual partners, and a history of sexual intercourse early in life. Because of their high risk, yearly Papanicolaou (Pap) smears are indicated. The practitioner should perform a pelvic examination and Pap smear if the client cannot remember where and when the last examination was done.

Yearly hemoccult testing of stool is indicated for adults 50 years of age or older. The practitioner should include a rectal examination and test for occult blood at each examination of a new patient older than 50 years of age, regardless of complaint.

Homeless adults are also at high risk for oropharyngeal cancer because of their frequent use of alcohol and cigarettes. The physical examination should include a careful examination of the oropharynx looking for leukoplakia.

Cholesterol Screening

Homeless adults usually have great difficulties eating an adequate diet, and measures to reduce cholesterol-rich foods may be virtually impossible. Nevertheless, a screening cholesterol test should still be performed on individuals who have additional risk factors for heart disease including coronary artery disease (especially if young), hypertension, diabetes, a family history of heart disease, or tobacco use. Screening will identify individuals who would benefit from cholesterol-reducing medications.

Glaucoma Screening

Glaucoma is highly prevalent in adults and a common cause of blindness. Risk factors for glaucoma include old age, male sex, black race, family history of glaucoma, diabetes, and hypertension. Early identification of glaucoma can prevent or minimize visual loss. Periodic tonometric screening should be conducted for homeless adults, particularly those with risk factors, after the age of 40.

Family Planning and Prenatal Care

Homeless health care providers should be knowledgeable about available birth control methods. They should provide birth control counseling to all homeless women of child-bearing age during all visits, even when homeless women are seen for unrelated problems. During these visits, women should be offered birth control, when available, or referred to local family planning facilities. Each contraceptive method has both advantages and disadvantages for the homeless woman. Oral contraceptives are problematic for smokers, and women with a substance abuse problem may forget to take them regularly. Additionally, the general chaos of a homeless woman's life may interfere with taking birth control pills daily. Thus, for many homeless women, the pill is probably not an ideal choice.

Barrier methods (condoms, diaphragms, etc.) have the advantages of fewer side effects than oral contraceptives and decreased risk of acquiring STDs, but the disadvantage of requiring patient compliance for proper use. The intrauterine device is probably the easiest and most effective contraceptive method for homeless women, but has become largely unavailable in the United States.

Given these realities, each homeless woman should be presented with contraceptive alternatives, the advantages and disadvantages of each method, and given whatever birth control method she is willing to use.

Routine and early prenatal care is critical to assure an optimal pregnancy outcome (see chapter 13 by McNally and Wood on obstetrical care for a detailed discussion of pregnancy care for homeless women).

HEALTH EVALUATION OF THE HOMELESS ADULT

Appointments or drop-in visits for acute medical problems are opportunities to address not only the presenting complaint, but also chronic conditions and preventive health needs. Underlying health conditions or needs may often be more serious than the specific problems for which an individual is seeking care. Homeless adults, with the daily problems they face, may focus only on the acute medical problems, however. For this reason, whenever possible, providers should include several preventive health screening measures during acute care clinic visits (see Table 5.1).

Medical History

Providers should ask if a homeless individual has had specific problem with each of the systems covered in a traditional "review of

Table 5.1 Preventive Health Screening Measures

History:
Past medical history
Preventive measures
Habits
Contraception, sexual, reproductive
Social
Family

Physical examination:
General appearance, blood pressure, skin, oropharynx, lymph nodes, lungs,
    heart, extremities, breast examination (especially if > 40 years), pelvic,
    rectal (adults > 50 years)

Laboratory procedures:
Tuberculosis screening yearly
Venereal Disease Research Laboratory (every 3–5 years)
Gonorrhea and chlamydia screening (yearly in sexually active women)
Pap (yearly)
Stool guaiac (yearly > 50 years)
Mammogram (yearly > 50 years; baseline 35–40 years)
Cholesterol (yearly, especially if high risk for heart disease)
HIV screening offered to high-risk individuals
Tonometry (every 3 years if > 40 years)

systems." This will uncover chronic conditions needing diagnosis or treatment, or identify specific health risk factors. In addition, a preventive health care history should be obtained. Unfortunately, many homeless patients will be unable to provide specific information. When taking the preventive health care history, providers should ask whether their patient has ever undergone a routine physical; had blood tests; or received screening tests for high blood pressure, tuberculosis, and STDs. An immunization history including the most recent tetanus booster, influenza, pneumovax, hepatitis B, and rubella vaccine for women of child-bearing age should also be obtained. In addition, practitioners should obtain a history about mental health problems, and drug, alcohol, and tobacco usage. Mental illness or substance abuse may significantly interfere with an individual's motivation to seek preventive health services or to follow through with prescribed regimens.

Clinicians should ask female patients (a) when they last received a breast and pelvic examination, and Pap smear; (b) whether or not they have a family history of breast cancer; (c) when and where they last had a mammogram; and (d) whether or not they are using birth control. Women should also be questioned about possible pregnancy.

Elderly patients should be specifically questioned about symptoms related to common cancers (e.g., weight loss, melena, etc.). If time permits, a dental and nutritional history should be obtained. To make the best use of the limited time available for examination, the provider can ask these questions while preforming a physical examination.

Social and Family Medical History

The practitioner should take a social history that includes information about housing, income, employment, job skills, social supports, and current stresses. Questions should be designed to elicit information about past and current living conditions. Is the individual receiving any income assistance? What is the individual's job history? Does he or she have particular work skills? Who does the client turn to during times of crisis? What is the nature of his or her support network?

This information not only bears directly on the health of the patient, but also gives the medical professional information on how best to manage the client's care and how to proceed with preventive medical care. For example, an individual who lives on the street has health needs that are different from someone who lives in a shelter where there are some supports. Shelter staff can facilitate clients' follow-up by reminding them of a health visit appointment, providing transportation, reading a tuberculin skin test, and so forth.

Although individuals often lack specific information about family history, it is still worth pursuing briefly. A family history of medical conditions, particularly hypertension, heart disease, diabetes, and some cancers place the individual at higher risk and indicate the need for additional screening measures.

Physical Examination

As discussed earlier, homeless health care providers should make use of appointments or drop-in visits for acute medical problems to address chronic medical problems and preventive health needs. During physical examination, practitioners should actively look for early signs or risk factors of treatable disease, especially those for which the homeless are at particular risk.

Screening for some medical problems can be done at the same time that the practitioner focuses on specific complaints. For example, the oropharynx can be inspected for precancerous and cancerous lesions when a sore throat is evaluated. Other screening measures will require the patient's consent. For instance, the practitioner will need to explain the reason for checking inguinal lymph nodes in an intravenous drug user who is at high risk for AIDS but only interested in curing a cough. In these instances, the practitioner might casually say: "Sometimes people have illnesses for a while before they notice them. As long as you are here for a cough, we may as well use this opportunity to check you for other kinds of problems. Is this OK with you?"

All examinations begin with observing the general appearance of the individual. This can usually be done while obtaining the history. Does the individual appear healthy? Do they look cachectic? Are they in any evident distress, either physical or emotional? Evidence of drug abuse (e.g., needle tracks, intoxication, suspiciousness, etc.) or mental illness (e.g., anxiety and restlessness, depression, signs of psychosis such as hallucination or delusions, etc.) should be noted. Vital signs should be taken, including weight and blood pressure, which should be checked for elevation. The skin can quickly be inspected for suspicious lesions. Careful examination of the oropharynx for evidence of white or red mucosal patches that may suggest cancer and dental problems can be done relatively quickly. Additional examination components should include palpation of lymph nodes, checking for tenderness or enlargement, which may indicate an STD, AIDS, or cancer, abdominal examination, palpating for organomegaly, liver or epigastric tenderness, masses, or ascites; cardiac and pulmonary auscultation, looking for evidence of pneumonia, congestive heart failure, or other abnormalities; and examination of the extremities, checking for signs of peripheral arterial disease (reduced or absent pulses, pallor on elevation, rubor on dependency), venous disease (varicosities, stasis changes, ulceration, swelling or edema), and cellulitis (erythema, swelling, streaking).

For all patients aged 50 or older, a rectal examination should be done to check for masses, blood in the stool, and the prostate in the male patient. A breast examination should be encouraged, particularly for women older than 40 years of age. A pelvic examination, Pap smear and cervical cultures should be performed yearly.

These intrusive parts of the examination will be more difficult to perform, particularly at outreach sites. Providers must develop rapport with the client and ensure privacy during the examination. Even then, clients may be unwilling to undergo a pelvic or rectal examination. In this case, providers should delay more sensitive parts of the examination until a trusting relationship has been established.

These recommendations comprise the minimum components of a preventive health examination. A complete examination would ideally include a thorough head, eyes, ears, nose, and throat evaluation, a neurological examination, and a testicular examination. Depending on the availability of time and the patient's willingness, all the elements of a complete examination may be included in one extended visit, or two or more shorter sessions.

Laboratory Procedures

In general, if an individual does not remember having had screening tests or recent immunizations, the provider should perform the indicated health screening test and administer the indicated immunizations. If an individual reports having had an intrusive or extensive procedure, such as a mammogram, HIV testing, or hepatitis vaccine, however, and can identify the provider, every effort should be made to retrieve the results. For example, rubella titers for young mothers can be requested from hospital records where their youngest child was delivered. The clinic should perform as many of the recommended preventive measures as the patient will tolerate. Tests should be prioritized, however, according to risk factors. For example, a mammogram is probably more important for a 60-year-old woman with a family history of breast cancer than are blood tests. Likewise, providing immunizations is especially important for individuals who are unlikely to receive follow-up care.

PREVENTIVE HEALTH PLAN

Providers should develop a simple preventive health plan for homeless adult patients based on age, gender, individual risk factors, and conditions commonly found among homeless adults. The plan should include preventive measures and health promotion interventions. For example, a woman of child-bearing age who is being evaluated for a cold should receive the following minimum preventive measures: a history that includes support system, health habits, contraception practice; and a brief examination that includes a breast and pelvic examination, Pap test, gonorrhea and chlamydia screening, tuberculosis and blood pressure screening, tetanus immunization, if indicated, and counseling regarding contraception, AIDS prevention, and nutrition. A summary of recommended baseline preventive measures is provided in Table 5.2.

Generally, the best approach to providing preventive services for homeless adults coordinates on-site clinic services with an effective outreach team. Linkage with clinic services is essential for those who are found to have any abnormalities. The outreach team can also encourage adults to go to a clinic for routine physicals and pelvic examinations, targeting individuals who are at greatest risk (e.g., pregnant mothers, alcoholics, intravenous drug users, persons taking medication, and elderly adults). The outreach team can refer adults to available health promotion and preventive services such as family planning agencies and dental care, and help adults follow-up with necessary appointments.

When an outside referral is necessary, prepare individuals by telling them about the potential obstacles and frustrations that lie ahead. At times outreach personnel can accompany a homeless individual to a referral visit. This may facilitate access to services and

Table 5.2 Preventive Health Guidelines for Homeless Adults

Immunizations:
Tetanus every 10 years
Influenza (yearly in high-risk persons[a])
Pneumovax (one time in high-risk persons[b])
Hepatitis B (given in three doses; high-risk persons[c])
Rubella

Educational topics that should be covered at outreach sites and clinics:
Family planning
Prenatal care
STD and AIDS prevention
Alcohol and drug abuse
Smoking
Nutrition
Hygiene
Dental care

[a]Persons with chronic cardiopulmonary disease, asthma, diabetes, immunosuppression. [b]All of the preceding, alcoholism, asplenia. [c]Intravenous drug users, homosexual men, sexual partners of these groups.

reduce the frustration of dealing with a new provider or bureaucratic health institution.

CONCLUSION

Preventive health care is not a high priority of homeless adults. This population, concerned with the present exigencies of their lives, seeks acute, episodic care. Thus, ensuring that the preventive health care needs of homeless persons are met is a challenge. A knowledge of conditions common among homeless adults, a realistic appraisal of how much preventive care can be provided during visits for acute problems, and a strong link between outreach teams and clinic staff increase the chance that homeless adults will receive necessary preventive health services.

REFERENCES

American Cancer Society. (1980). Report on the cancer-related health check-up. *Cancer 30*, 194–240.

Canadian Task Force on the Periodic Health Examination. (1984). The periodic health examination, 1984 update. *Canadian Medical Association Journal, 130*, 1278.

Wright J. D., & Weber, E. (1987). *Homelessness and Health*. New York: McGraw-Hill.

Adult Medical Issues

Chronic Disease in the Homeless

6

Susan Fleischman, Tom Farnham

CHAPTER HIGHLIGHTS

- Studies have found that 30% to 40% of the homeless suffer from one or more chronic health problems.
- Chronic diseases among the homeless are typically long-standing, untreated, and of greater severity than in the domiciled population.
- The stress of homelessness, exposure to the elements, and personal problems such as alcohol, drug, or tobacco abuse make the management of chronic disease in the homeless populatiom complex and frustrating.
- All homeless patients, no matter what their presenting complaint, should be screened for chronic health problems.
- Chronic conditions commonly found in the homeless population include hypertension, diabetes, peripheral vascular disease, chronic obstructive pulmonary disease, heart disease, and seizures.
- Standard textbook recommendations for treatment of chronic diseases are often unreasonable and unrealistic in the homeless setting.
- Successful treatment of chronic illness requires creative new approaches tailored to the disease and the homeless setting; these include the use of outreach teams, public health nurses, frequent work.

79

INTRODUCTION

The prevalence of chronic illness among homeless adults is much higher than in the general population. In a Los Angeles survey of homeless adults, 40 percent reported at least one chronic health problem (Ropers & Boyer, 1987).

Among the homeless adults served by the 19-city Robert Wood Johnson homeless health care project, clinics reported that 31% of clients had one or more chronic physical disorders (Wright, 1987). More than 40% of clients seen in the clinics more than once had at least one chronic disease. The most common chronic diseases diagnosed among homeless adults are hypertension and heart disease, peripheral vascular disease, chronic obstructive pulmonary disease, diabetes, dental problems, and neurological disorders.

Several factors combine to explain this high prevalence of chronic disease. First, life-style factors common among homeless persons, such as alcohol, drug, and tobacco use are all risk factors for cardiovascular disease and other chronic illness. For example, hypertension is twice as common among heavy drinkers than among nondrinkers. (Wright, 1987). Second, once homeless, exposure to the elements, nutritional deficiencies, and victimization can worsen existing chronic illness. Third, chronic illness itself can limit a person's ability to work, and lead to impoverishment and even homelessness. Lastly, the increased incidence of chronic disease among homeless adults may be due, in part, to a history of inadequate access to health services, especially preventive care. Homeless persons experience many barriers to health care (see Chapter 2 by Koegel and Gelberg) including lack of health insurance, medical providers' reluctance to see homeless persons, and the daily demands of finding food and shelter that characterize the homeless life-style. Attending to chronic health problems or seeking preventive care may be low priority in this setting.

In this chapter, we limit our discussion to the commonest chronic diseases seen among the homeless: hypertension, diabetes, peripheral vascular disease, chronic obstructive pulmonary disease, cardiac disease including angina and congestive heart failure, and seizures.

ASSESSMENT

Chronic illnesses may be silent, without manifestations until late in their course. Because of limited medical attention, chronic problems among the homeless often go unrecognized and untreated, resulting in high levels of morbidity and mortality. Moreover, even with detection and treatment, compliance problems among the homeless often result in unabated progression of the disease, disability, morbidity, and premature death.

Generally, adults tend to seek care for specific, episodic health care problems or symptoms. This is especially true of the homeless. Because of their survival needs, homeless adults will often not present to the clinic until symptoms seriously affect their life-style. When they present with a relatively minor acute health problem, they may not even mention the existence of a serious chronic illness. Because of the high prevalence of chronic undiagnosed illness, all homeless patients, regardless of their chief complaint, should be screened for hypertension with a blood pressure check, for diabetes and renal disease with a routine urinalysis (for glucose and protein), and, if possible, for anemia with a hemoglobin or hematocrit. Intake assessments should include blood pressure, heart rate, respiratory rate, temperature, and weight, if possible. This should be followed by as complete a physical examination as is possible, and a routine urinalysis and hematocrit.

Often these initial screening examinations are done by outreach teams (see chapter 4 Smith on outreach). Patients with an abnormal screening examination should be referred to the central clinic for full evaluation. In addition to a full history and physical, laboratory tests that may be necessary are listed in Table 6.1. Of course, the central clinic may not have the ability to perform many of these laboratory tests. Therefore, a referral network that allows easy referral and ready follow-up of homeless clients is needed for further evaluations.

HYPERTENSION

Diagnosis

Screening programs among homeless adults have found abnormally high blood pressure in one quarter to one third of clients screened (Wright, 1987). Ropers and Boyer (1987) found that 39% of the homeless reported a history of hypertension. Another study found a prevalence of 60% among older residents of SRO facilities, whereas the prevalence in shelters was found to be 28% (Kellog, 1985). Hypertension is twice as prevalent in alcoholics than in nonalcoholics. Hypertension may be asymptomatic and found on routine

Table 6.1 Appropriate Laboratory Tests to Evaluate Abnormalities in Screening

Screening test	Follow-up laboratory test indicated
Elevated blood pressure	Sodium, potassium chloride, bicarbonate
	Creatinine
	EKG
	Chest radiograph (if clinically indicated; see text)
Urinalysis positive for glucose	Blood glucose
Urinalysis positive for protein	Microscopic urinalysis
	Creatinine
	Twenty-four-hour urine for protein, and creatinine clearance (if indicated)
Urinalysis positive—white blood cells or nitrate	Microscopic urinalysis
	Urine culture
Abnormal hemoglobin	Complete blood count
	Iron studies
	Serum B_{12} and folate levels
	Stool testing for occult blood, if indicated

screening, or present with symptoms of headache, dizziness, chest pain, shortness of breath, and, rarely, gross hematuria. Frequently, homeless patients have been previously diagnosed for hypertension, but may not have taken medication for months or years.

When evaluating a patient for hypertension, the history should include questions regarding a family history of hypertension, alcohol use, and prior diagnosis or treatment of hypertension. The evaluation should include a complete physical examination, baseline laboratory examinations of serum creatinine and potassium, routine urinalysis, and EKG. The presence of left ventricular hypertrophy on EKG may indicate that the hypertension has been present for longer than suspected. Evidence of ischemia or an old myocardial infarction on EKG indicates the presence of coronary artery disease.

Treatment

For nonemergent hypertension, diagnosis and possible treatment should be considered at the first visit. In the homeless, for whom follow-up is poor, the traditional recommendation of multiple blood pressure determinations before treatment is impractical. Similarly, the recommendation to begin treatment with dietary changes is futile. Food at shelters and in soup lines is high in sodium and fat.

Thresholds for starting drug therapy must be individualized, considering diminished compliance, poor follow-up, and compounding life-style variables, such as alcohol abuse. In homeless alcoholics with hypertension, referral for alcohol detoxification may be a more appropriate treatment than drug therapy for the hypertension.

For those who require drug intervention, the ideal drug should incorporate the following considerations: once-daily dosing, limited need for laboratory follow-up (i.e., avoid potassium-losing diuretics), and no rebound phenomenon (because poor compliance and lost medications may precipitate this complication). Appropriate beginning regimens could be from one of the following category of medications: a potassium-sparing diuretic, a long-acting beta blocker, a long-acting calcium channel blocker, or a central-acting agent that does not cause rebound hypertension when abruptly discontinued. Additionally, medications should be dispensed free of charge, on-site, and in sufficient quantity to last until the next visit. Owing to the frequency of lost medication, a mechanism for easy replacement should be established.

Patient education is the key to compliance. Taking daily medication for a silent illness may be low priority for homeless patients. As the following case study illustrates, it may take months of education and follow-up before a homeless patient is willing to follow a treatment regimen.

A 52-year-old homeless man has long-standing hypertension and a questionable history of alcohol abuse. He was repeatedly noncompliant and would not take his blood pressure medication or show up for clinic visits. When he did show up at the clinic, usually with extremely high blood pressure, he was accommodated on a walk-in basis. At each visit, he was again given medication and educated regarding compliance. Unfortunately he was then lost to follow-up and presented again 6 months later having suffered a stroke. He was no longer using alcohol. He was again restarted on blood pressure medications and told that he might prevent further strokes by taking his medication. He now comes to the clinic weekly for medications and has a clearer understanding of his illness. This would not have occurred without the clinic's frequent intervention.

Initially, patients should be seen as frequently as every several days after initiating therapy to evaluate compliance and efficacy. Patients should be advised that decreasing salt, calories, and alcohol ingestion would be helpful, but this should not be the mainstay of therapy.

Malignant hypertension manifested by increased blood pressure and mental status changes, stroke, chest pain, or vision changes should be managed as a medical emergency. Medications, such as nifedipine or clonidine, should be given to reduce blood pressure immediately, and the paramedics should be called to transport the patient to the closest emergency department.

DIABETES

Diagnosis

All homeless patients should be screened for diabetes by a routine urinalysis. Glycosuria should be evaluated with a capillary blood sugar determination. If the homeless patient currently has symptoms consistent with diabetes, has a history of diabetes in the past, or a family history of diabetes, a capillary blood glucose should be evaluated. Presenting complaints may range from the typical polyuria, polydipsia, and blurred vision to diabetic-related infections or complications such as candidiasis, bronchitis, skin infections, and foot and leg ulcers.

The physical examination should include a search for evidence of retinopathy, neuropathy, and peripheral vascular changes. The feet should be carefully examined for neuropathy, vascular changes and ulcers. Footwear should be inspected and replaced if it could potentially cause problems. The laboratory evaluation should include a urinalysis for glucose and protein, capillary blood glucose, a serum creatinine, and electrolytes and an EKG to screen for heart disease.

Treatment

The decision to initiate treatment of homeless diabetics must take into consideration their environment, life-style, comorbid diseases, and addictions. Strict adherence to the American Diabetic Association guidelines for diagnosis and treatment is not possible. The thresholds for the initiation of therapy depend not only on the patient's blood sugar, but also on his or her living situation. Limited access to food is the major limiting variable in treatment. Even in the best shelters, round-the-clock access to food, in the event of hypoglycemia, is not possible. This problem is worse for those on the street who depend on food lines; it is still worse for the alcohol-dependent homeless individuals who may never follow a regular diet. Because of these and other limitations, the goal of therapy cannot be tight control of blood glucose. As in the case of hypertension, dietary changes should not be the mainstay of therapy. Oral hypoglycemics are the safest treatment in this setting. The goal is moderate control of blood glucose without hypoglycemia.

Because of the extreme danger of hypoglycemia, only rarely should insulin be considered. Other problems with insulin therapy include lack of storage for insulin, needles, and syringes, and finding a clean site for injection. Insulin therapy should be limited to either ketosis-prone or severely hyperglycemic patients. The goals of therapy should be very loose control. This is most simply and safely accomplished using once- or twice-daily doses of NPH intermediate-acting insulin.

The following case study demonstrates the need for flexibility and accommodation when making medical decisions regarding treatment of homeless diabetic patients.

A 45-year-old woman with below-average intelligence has been homeless for many years. She most recently has been living at a local church shelter. When she was seen at the clinic with multiple skin infections and vaginal candidiasis, a diagnosis of diabetes was made. The patient's blood sugars were originally moderately controlled with oral medication. As her diet worsened and her weight increased, however, her glucose became extremely high. With the help of another homeless client who lives at the same shelter, this women was started on once-daily low-dose insulin injections, given to her by the other client. We were unable to increase to twice-daily injections because the other client was not available at the shelter in the afternoon. Working with a social service agency, a board and care facility was found that would take the woman and administer her insulin twice daily.

Follow-up should be biweekly or more frequently until the patient's blood sugar and insulin regimen are stabilized. Education concerning hypoglycemia, proper foot care, and symptoms of severely uncontrolled blood sugar should be done at each visit. Podiatry and ophthalmology referrals should be made at least once soon after diagnosis for formal evaluations. Referral for hospitalization should be considered at a lower clinical threshold for the homeless than for the domiciled or nondiabetic patient.

PERIPHERAL VASCULAR DISEASE

Diagnosis

Peripheral vascular disease (PVD) includes a broad group of illnesses including chronic edema, lower extremity cellulitis, and phlebitis. All of these frequently derive from venous or arterial insufficiency. The prevalences of these conditions in the homeless are 10 to 15 times greater than in the general population (Wright & Weber, 1987). Brickner (1973) reported a 10% incidence of leg ulcers or cellulitis in the homeless. The inordinately high rate of PVD among the homeless is the direct result of life-style: constant walking, the inability to elevate the legs during sleep, poor hygiene, and exposure are all etiological factors in PVD.

Patients may present with chronic statis ulcerations, stasis dermatitis or only pedal edema. Ulceration is most commonly found around the medial malleolus but may occur in other pressure point areas. The skin ulcerations are frequently complicated by infection. The physical examination should look for signs of heart failure, renal disease, or other causes of pedal edema. Diabetes and renal disease can be screened for with a routine urinalysis.

Treatment

The most important intervention for PVD is a change in life-style. Elevation of legs, at least during sleep, is the key to treatment. A network of shelter referrals for beds (not pews), respite beds, or hotel vouchers may be required if the clinic is to help the homeless client find a place to elevate his or her legs. Bus tokens should be given to limit the need for walking long distances.

For patients with ulcers, daily cleaning and dressing of the wound is the most effective therapy, even if it requires daily clinic visits. Wounds that appear infected require oral antibiotics in addition to local care. Dressing materials, sufficient for several wound changes, should be given to the homeless client. Ace wraps are helpful to protect the wound and compress the veins, reducing blood stasis. External compression stockings and proper footwear are also necessary for ongoing prevention. Appropriate foot care and wound care are especially important in the homeless diabetic with vascular disease. Hospital referral should be considered for cellulitis or severe nonhealing ulcers. Longer-term therapy may require board-and-care placement or other long-term housing placement.

CHRONIC OBSTRUCTIVE PULMONARY DISEASE

Diagnosis

The Robert Wood Johnson homeless project found a 5% prevalence of COPD (chronic obstructive pulmonary disease) in the homeless. Much of this is probably tobacco associated. Presenting complaints include shortness of breath, wheezing, dyspnea on exertion, decreased exercise tolerance, or chronic cough. The physical examination should include a peak flow measurement. This can be done simply with a "Wright" peak flow meter, even at outreach sites. A chest radiograph should be obtained if wheezing is localized, rather than diffuse, or when making a new diagnosis of COPD. Pulmonary function tests are helpful to clarify the diagnosis of COPD or to assess severity.

Treatment

Traditional management of COPD includes the use of systemic theophyline, inhaled beta adrenergics, steroids, and curtailment of smoking. In our experience in treating the homeless, only inhaled beta adrenergics, because of the immediate relief they provide, are used regularly. Exacerbations can be treated in the clinic setting with nebulized beta adrenergics. Antibiotics should be used liberally with exacerbations, but patients should be carefully monitored for drug interactions such as the potentiation of theophylline by erythromycin. Many patients may also require oral steroids. Steroid therapy initially requires daily evaluation.

Because adults with COPD are at risk for serious pneumococcal pneumonia or influenza, pneumovax and yearly influenza vaccination should be administered to all homeless adults with a diagnosis of COPD or a smoking history greater than 30 pack-years.

HEART DISEASE

Diagnosis

The actual incidence of heart disease among homeless adults is unknown but estimates range from 2.9% (Ropers & Boyer, 1987) to 10% to 15% (Brickner & Kauffman,1973). Heart disease is particularly common among older homeless patients, especially those with long-standing, possibly untreated, hypertension. Smoking and alcohol abuse are comorbid risk factors that greatly increase the likelihood of heart disease.

Screening for heart disease consists of questioning all older patients for symptoms of angina and congestive heart failure. This should also be done for all patients found to have hypertension, diabetes, or other vascular disease. Symptoms can range from mild decreased exertional capacity such as difficulty going upstairs to shortness of breath at rest. Questions should probe for recent dramatic weight gain, swollen legs, or tight shoes. Nighttime symptoms such as orthopnea, paroxysmal nocturnal dyspnea, or even nocturia may be difficult to determine in a client who only sleeps episodically. Direct questions exploring for the presence of anginal symptoms should be part of the interview. The clinician should ask about typical exertional chest pain and also less typical angina presentations such as shortness of breath on exertion.

Physical findings may be subtle and limited. Angina alone may not produce physical findings, and clinicians should look for other clues to the presence of atherosclerotic vascular disease: eyegrounds should be examined for vascular changes, and the neck, abdomen, and groin ausculated for bruits. The cardiac examination should evaluate the point of maximal impulse for cardiomegaly, and auscultate for gallops or murmurs, indicating possible valvular disease or heart failure. The lung examination may be obscured by concomitant COPD from tobacco abuse. Nonetheless, rales and other signs of congestion may indicate congestive heart failure. The presence of pedal edema may be due to venous disease rather than cardiac disease and is not helpful in making the diagnosis of congestive heart failure.

The laboratory evaluation will vary depending on the clinic and availability of referral resources. All patients with suspected heart disease should have at least an EKG to assess for chamber enlargement or the presence of an old myocardial infarction. A chest radiograph can help elucidate heart size as well as evaluate lung changes consistent with heart failure or lung disease. The decision to pursue a more extensive evaluation such as exercise treadmill, echocardiography, or holter monitoring will depend on the individual patient's level of impairment because of heart disease, and results of the EKG and chest radiograph.

Treatment

Treatment of heart disease in homeless adults is quite difficult. The mainstay of therapy for angina remains nitrates, beta blockers, and calcium channel blockers. New bottles of sublingual nitroglycerin should be provided liberally. The treatment of heart failure is complicated by the high risk of complication from medications. High-dose diuretics, digoxin, and antiarrhytyhmics cannot be used without frequent or daily follow-up visits and multiple laboratory evaluations.

Homeless persons may need to be admitted more often to the hospital and at a lower clinical threshold than the domiciled population. For example, controlling sodium intake and enforcing bedrest, mainstays of therapy in the domiciled population, are virtually impossible in the homeless. Hospitalization is often required to achieve adequate diuresis in a controlled environment where electrolytes can be monitored.

SEIZURES

Seizures, with an incidence of approximately 4% (Roper & Boyer, 1987), are the most common neurological illness found in the homeless. The most common causes of seizures in this population are first alcohol abuse followed by head trauma.

Diagnosis

Patients who present with new episodes of loss of consciousness require a work-up to rule out causes other than alcohol, such as cardiac arrhythmias or trauma. Patients presenting with a seizure for the first time require an electroencephalogram (EEG), a metabolic work-up, as well as a head computed axial tomographic scan to rule out a mass lesion.

Most seizure patients present with a long history of frequent, witnessed seizures and multiple subsequent emergency department visits. Patients who present with a past history of seizures may actually be more difficult to assess and treat than the patient with new-onset seizures. Because treatments differ, it is important to separate patients who have strictly alcohol-related seizures from those whose seizures are caused by other factors. A clear history of seizures limited to times of heavy alcohol use or withdrawal is helpful. Likewise, a lack of seizures during long periods of sobriety is helpful in making a diagnosis of alcohol-related seizures. Alcoholics are also at high risk for serious or recurrent head trauma, however. A seizure that appears to be alcohol related by history, may in fact be due to acute or chronic head trauma. The EEG is helpful in making this distinction; simple, alcohol related seizures show generalized, nonfocal changes on EEG, whereas an EEG in seizures owing to trauma or intracranial hemorrhage usually has focal findings. This distinction is often difficult to sort out, however.

Treatment

Treatment will depend on the etiologic classification of the seizures as well as the natural history of seizures in the patient. Although there is clear evidence that phenytoin is not useful in alcohol-related seizures, most emergency departments still discharge alcoholics with prescriptions for phenytoin. Alcoholics who have a seizure from alcohol withdrawal are more appropriately treated by referral to an inpatient medical detoxification facility. Similarly, outpatient treatment with benzodiazepines in an alcoholic is fraught with possible complications such as drug interactions with alcohol, benzodiazepine abuse, and overdose.

In those individuals with seizures not clearly related to alcohol use, appropriate drug choices are similar to those used in domiciled patients. Patients should be seen often to monitor for side effects of anticonvulsants as well as to have medication levels checked. As with other chronic illnesses in the homeless, compliance and follow-up issues complicate and compromise care.

CONCLUSION

The homeless have an increased incidence of chronic illnesses, especially hypertension and peripheral vascular disease. These may be caused or exacerbated by the homeless life-style. Because of lack of preventive and continuous health care, chronic disease in the homeless is often detected late, making successful intervention difficult. Standard textbook recommendations for treatment are unreasonable and unrealistic in this setting. Creative new approaches using frequent clinic visits, outreach teams, public health nurses, and social service networking are required for successful treatment.

REFERENCES

Brickner, K., & Kaufman, (1973). Case findings of heart diseases in homeless men. *Bulletin of the New York Academy of Medicine, 49*(6): 475–484.

Kellogg, R. (1985). Hypertension—A screening and treatment program for the homeless. In K. Brickner (Ed.), *Health care of Homeless People* (Vol. 8, pp. 109-119).

Ropers, R., Boyer, R. (1987, Spring). Homeless as a health risk. *Alcohol Health and Research World,* 11 pgs 38-41.

Wright, J., & Weber E., Homelessness and health. New York: McGraw-Hill.

Management of Substance Abuse in Primary Care Setting

James R. Lockyer

7

CHAPTER HIGHLIGHTS

- Homeless adults are particularly susceptible to intravenous drug, alcohol, and cocaine abuse.
- Denial, fear of being turned away from shelters or other services, or underlying psychiatric problems make it difficult to obtain an accurate history of substance abuse.
- To help homeless substance abusers, clinicians should follow the "four C's" approach: convenience, confidentiality, compassion, and community.
- Learning which drugs are used in different homeless communities and which drugs are currently on the street will help with diagnosis, patient communication, and treatment.
- Homeless health care providers should be expert in the signs and symptoms of acute intoxication and chronic use, the means of administration, complications of alcohol or drug abuse, and even the local drug culture and slang terminology used on the streets.
- The provider must be sensitive to the patient's willingness and ability to accept treatment.
- The assessment and treatment of alcohol, cocaine, and intravenous drug abuse among the homeless are presented.

INTRODUCTION

Drug and alcohol abuse are epidemic in the United States. Alcohol abuse alone is responsible for the annual loss of approximately 350,000 lives, and alcohol-related illnesses account for as much as 40% of all hospitalizations in the United States (Wright et al., 1987).

More than 500,000 Americans are estimated to be intravenous drug users (IVDUs). The practice of injecting drugs under unsterile conditions has a profound impact on the health of its victims. It also serves as a major source for transmission of infectious diseases into the general population. Presently, the second most significant single risk factor for AIDS is IVDU; 17% of people with AIDS are IVDUs. Projections suggest that, with the modification of high-risk behavior among the homosexual population, intravenous drug users and their sexual partners will make up an increasing share of the AIDS population.

Homeless adults and the skid row inhabitants are particularly susceptible to intravenous drug abuse and alcohol abuse. Moreover, introduction of more potent, accessible forms of cocaine (free-basing, crack) has resulted in a dramatic increase in drug use in the general population and among the homeless in particular. Last year alone, cocaine toxicity caused an estimated 3,000 deaths nationwide.

According to one survey, almost 60% of the adult homeless population used alcohol or illicit drugs on a regular basis (Brickner, 1985). Alcohol and drug abuse among parents in homeless families is also quite high at 30% to 40%. Drug and alcohol abuse imposes a tremendous burden on the health and welfare of persons in the homeless setting, causing increased morbidity and mortality owing to heart disease, neurological disease, traumatic injury, infectious diseases, psychiatric disorders, and malnutrition (Wright et al., 1987).

A multidisciplinary approach is needed to cope with the complexity of drug and alcohol abuse among the homeless. Psychological, economic, social, and medical factors must be considered in addressing the problem. The following discussion focuses on the recognition and treatment of alcoholism and substance abuse in the homeless population.

GENERAL CONSIDERATIONS FOR THE EVALUATION AND MANAGEMENT OF SUBSTANCE ABUSE

Substance abusers frequently pose unique and difficult challenges to the clinician. Persons using alcohol or street drugs often exhibit a significant degree of denial; getting them to recognize their problem is a major first step. They may also be extremely reluctant, out of paranoia or a fear of legal prosecution, to provide an accurate history of their substance abuse. IVDUs often have underlying psychiatric problems including paranoid delusions, psychosis, or passive-aggressive personality disorders, which further complicate history taking and management. To cope effectively with the challenge of assisting substance abusers, we follow the "four C's" approach: convenience, confidentiality, compassion, and community.

Convenience

The life-style of most substance abusers revolves around their addiction. The alcoholic will start his day with a drink to "stop the shakes." Heroin or cocaine addicts will focus their daily routine around procurement and use of drugs. Consequently, concerns such as health, adequate clothing, and general welfare assume a lower priority. Substance abusers are often reluctant to seek assistance for medical problems because long bus rides to a clinic and lengthy waits interfere with their substance abuse activities.

To help substance abusers effectively, the medical facility must be centrally located and convenient to the population it serves. The registration process should be brief and waiting times kept to a minimum. Compliance with follow-up visits in the substance abuse population is notoriously poor, making it important to assess patients comprehensively at each encounter. Obtain all indicated laboratory studies at the initial visit. Provide medications in a format that ensures a balance between a comprehensive therapeutic regimen and maximum ease in dosing (e.g., administration twice a day instead of three times a day).

Throughout the registration, evaluation, and treatment, health workers should use each available moment to emphasize the potential dangers of substance abuse, the need for safer sex practices such as condom use, and the avoidance of needle sharing.

Confidentiality

For obvious reasons, substance abusers are much less likely to use a health care facility if they are concerned about the confidentiality of their visit. Often their perceptions may be a manifestation of paranoia, making it important for the health team to be overly cautious in this regard. Providers should make a special effort to reassure nervous patients concerning confidentiality. It is not enough to say, "the information you give me is confidential." Patients who abuse drugs may not know what you mean. Providers need to be very specific in their discussion of confidentiality. We tell our patients that, "the police will have nothing to do with this, and I will not tell your SRO operator. These are your medical records and no one outside the clinic is allowed to look at them."

A substance abuser is more inclined to confide in the clinician if he or she believes that the provider has a realistic appreciation of the patient's predicament. The more in-depth the provider's comprehension of the situation, the more likely the patient will be to trust him or her. A clinician's knowledge of current slang, and drug prices and practices in the area helps to gain the patient's confidence. Once a relationship has been established, the patient will be more receptive to counseling, have better compliance with therapeutic regimens, and be more open to rehabilitation.

Compassion

All interaction should be in a warm, professional manner, void of judgmental attitudes or behavior. Information regarding the dangers of alcohol or drug abuse must be provided in a direct, matter-of-fact manner. Moralizing and self-righteousness will only alienate the addict and eliminate all hope of communicating effectively.

Community

To treat substance abuse among the homeless effectively, clinicians need to be familiar with the community in which the homeless live. For example, finding out where a patient "hangs out" provides valuable clues as to his or her addiction. In the skid row area of Los Angeles, for example, patients who hang out by the "Wall," an area around San Julian and Wall Street in downtown Los Angeles, are likely to use cocaine. Those who congregate at a particular skid row hotel are more likely to be intravenous drug users. Phencyclidine piperdine (PCP) is typically found in East Los Angeles and an area of South Central Los Angeles known as "Sherman Way" (for the "sherms" that are smoked).

As a part of our effort to keep abreast of what's happening in the community, the clinic maintains close contact with the police department. This contact provides the clinic with information on what drugs are currently on the street. For example, the police recently notified us that they were seeing a purer form of heroin—30%, instead of the usual 5%. Because of this information, the clinic stocked extra naloxone hydrochloride (Narcan), an antidote for heroin overdose.

Working with homeless patients who abuse alcohol or drugs requires patience along with the four "C's." As the following case study illustrates, however, the time and effort spent with these patients sometimes pays off:

> A 32-year-old black woman initially presented to our medical facility in the Los Angeles skid row district more than a year ago. She had recently moved from Louisiana hoping to find employment.
>
> At her initial visit to the clinic, this woman was markedly hypertensive (170/120 mm Hg), without evidence of malignant changes. Although she would not take her hypertensive medication, she occasionally came to the clinic for acute care problems. At one clinic visit, her physical signs suggested acute narcotic intoxication: her blood pressure was normal for the first time (140/86 mm Hg), an indication of heroin use, and her pupils were miotic. When questioned about possible drug use, she finally admitted that her new boyfriend, a crack cocaine and intravenous heroin user, had talked her into trying heroin.
>
> At my urging, this woman came to the clinic more often, sometimes just for a social visit. Eventually, as her boyfriend became increasingly abusive, she began to consider giving up heroin and leaving her boyfriend. Finally, after several beatings, she consented to transitional housing arranged by the clinic. Daily clinic visits helped her cope with mild heroin withdrawal and served as a source of encouragement to avoid relapse.
>
> This woman developed a relationship with another man who was similarly homeless. They decided that, if they were ever to improve their situation, they needed to leave Los Angeles. Our clinic paid their bus fare back to Louisiana.

Through follow-up telephone calls and letters, we learned that this woman was accepted back by her family. She and her boyfriend married, and he has recently completed a job-training course as a truck driver. This woman began taking her medicine, and her blood pressure is now adequately controlled.

ALCOHOL ABUSE

Assessment

Most studies indicate that approximately 45% of the adult homeless males and 15% of adult homeless female population abuse alcohol on a regular basis (Wright et al., 1987).

Alcohol consumption has a profound impact on the health and safety of both the male and female homeless population because of its multiple acute and chronic adverse effects. When acutely inebriated, the homeless person is less capable of defending himself or herself against attack or sexual assault, and cannot appreciate the presence or severity of injuries or infections, which occur as a matter of routine while living on the street. Furthermore, the vasodilation induced by acute ethanol consumption increases heat loss and susceptibility to hypothermia.

Chronic ethanol consumption is toxic to virtually every organ system, and results in an array of abnormalities that often become life threatening. Several common or more significant sequelae of chronic alcohol consumption are listed in Table 7.1. This list is only partial, and is provided primarily to demonstrate the range of organ systems and the varied symptoms, signs, and comorbid conditions associated with chronic alcoholism.

The staggering gait and impaired sensorium that typify a person under the influence of alcohol are familiar to most of us. The possibility of other etiologies such as a traumatic subdural hematoma, tuberculous meningitis, or diabetic ketoacidosis, in which the patient has a "fruity" ketone breath and impaired mental status, must also be considered, however. Mild hypothermia (see chapter 11 by Lockyer on hypothermia) may also simulate alcohol intoxication with dysarthria, an ataxic gait, and an impaired level of consciousness. If any of these conditions are present *and* the homeless person ingested alcohol recently, the clinical picture may be truly confusing.

Table 7.1 Pathological Conditions Associated With Chronic Ethanol Consumption

Alcoholic liver disease
Cirrhosis
Pancreatitis
Alcoholic gastritis
Peptic ulcer disease
Esophageal carcinoma
Mallory-Weiss esophageal variceal tears and hemorrhages
Portal hypertension
Esophageal varices
Nutritional deficiencies (B_{12}, folate, thiamine)
Thrombocytopenia
Alcoholic neuropathy
Coagulopathy
Subdural hematoma
Dementia
Wernicke-Kosakoff's psychosis
Tuberculosis
Delirium tremens

History and Clinical Manifestations

Patients should be quickly evaluated for the commonest causes of an impaired sensorium through a brief but comprehensive history. Often companions or shelter staff can provide an adequate history and help to establish the diagnosis. The clinician should illicit a thorough history of the patient's drinking habit during the physical examination.

A standardized history to assess the level of alcohol abuse is not useful for the homeless. Questions about whether the patient is often late for work or been arrested while driving under the influence are not appropriate because homeless alcoholics have neither jobs or cars. Usually, however, it is not difficult to spot homeless alcoholics, most of whom are drunk all day and come to the clinic inebriated. Homeless alcoholics do not usually deny their addiction and will respond truthfully if asked directly about their drinking habits.

Typically, a person who is acutely intoxicated will be plethoric from peripheral vasodilation and may exhibit a mild tachycardia, moderate hypertension, and a low-grade temperature elevation. Sclerae are often injected.

Many common health problems of homeless adults are complicated by alcoholism: traumatic injuries bleed more easily and heal more slowly; seizures are often due to alcoholism or may be worsened by alcohol consumption; skin diseases, such as stasis ulcers, are commoner and difficult to treat; and hypertension and its side effects are exacerbated.

Evidence of long-standing alcoholism is exhibited primarily by the stigmata of liver disease. Findings include parotid gland hypertrophy, spider telangiectasia, gynecomastia, jaundice, ascites, pedal edema, and easy bruisability. Tremor, lateral nystagmus, and confabulation may also be signs of alcoholism. Many of these physical findings appear only after years of alcohol abuse. If few signs are present, the clinician must rely on an accurate history of the patient's behavior and drinking habits in making the diagnosis of ethanol abuse.

Laboratory Assessment

Several of laboratory tests are abnormal because of acute and chronic alcohol consumption. Table 7.2 lists many of the commoner or more significant laboratory abnormalities.

Our policy in the skid row clinic is to limit laboratory tests to those indicated to evaluate the presenting problem or specific symptomatic conditions. We do not routinely use laboratory examinations to screen for other problems. We have found, for example, that it is not cost effective to screen asymptomatic alcoholics for anemia, liver disease or other conditions because follow-up is extremely poor.

When, however, the patient presents with symptoms related to complications of alcoholism, we will perform the laboratory examinations indicated. For instance, if the patient has signs of a bleeding disorder (e.g., multiple bruises, petechiae, bleeding episodes, black stools, or they have thrown up blood), then we perform a complete blood count, platelet count, prothrombin time, partial prothrombin time, bleeding time, and other tests as needed.

Our clinic also performs all the laboratory tests listed in Table 7.2 for all patients entering a treatment program. When alcoholic patients come to the clinic, we emphasize the need for a rehabilitation program. The clinic provides them with a list of programs and tells them that we will do everything we can to help them get into a program when they are ready. Only when alcoholic patients are enrolled in a rehabilitation program can we effectively treat them for

Table 7.2 Laboratory Abnormalities Associated With Ingestion of Ethanol

Laboratory parameter	Considerations
Liver function tests:	
Increased SGOT (AST) Increased SGPT (ALT)	Alcoholic liver disease, alcoholic hepatitis, or cirrhosis; in chronic alcohol abuse, usually a low-grade elevation of liver function tests with a SGOT/SGPT ration of 2:1
Increased bilirubin Increased LDH	Laennec's cirrhosis or alcoholic hepatitis.
Complete blood count:	
Microcytic Anemia	Chronic gastrointestinal hemorrhage
Macrocytic anemia or macrocytosis	B_{12} or folate deficiency; may also be due to impaired red-cell membrane synthesis from liver disease
Thrombocytopenia	Marrow suppression versus splenic sequestration
Other Tests:	
Elevated creatinine phosphokinase	Rhabdomyolysis
Elevated amylase	Acute or subacute pancreatitis

Note. SGOT = serum glatamic = oxaloacetic transaminase; SGPT = serum glutamic = pyruvic transaminase; AST = aspartate aminotransferase; ALT = alanine aminotransferase; LDH = lactate dehydrogenase.

such serious complications of alcoholism as anemia and liver dysfunction.

Treatment

The homeless alcoholic patient is typically more interested in his addiction than in his health and is, consequently, more likely to come to a medical facility only when an acute event occurs. Therefore, we use the clinic visit as an opportunity to perform needed preventive care. Alcoholic patients should be assessed for tetanus vaccination status, and given a yearly screening for tuberculosis (PPD skin test or chest radiographs). The patient should be offered vitamin supplements, including thiamine and folate, whenever possible. Also, during clinic visits, efforts should be made to ensure that adequate food, clothing, and shelter are available to the alcoholic patient.

Wound care and injections require an aggressive approach because of impaired wound healing in alcoholic patients. These patients should be encouraged to return to the clinic for bandage changes or routine follow-up on a daily basis. Frequent clinic visits provide the opportunity to discuss more long-term assistance for the patient's problem, such as entry into a rehabilitation program.

Acute intoxication with alcohol is usually a self-limited phenomenon that requires no intervention. Evidence of dehydration should be treated with appropriate measures. If the person has an impaired sensorium, then it is essential to rule out possible coexistent problems such as a subdural hematoma, turberculous meningitis, or hypothermia.

Aspiration pneumonia is particularly common among skid row alcoholics. It is typically manifested by a right, middle, or lower lobe infiltrate that oftentimes contain anaerobic organisms from the oral cavity that are prone to abscess formation.

Alcohol withdrawal, if untreated, imposes a 15% to 20% mortality rate. With appropriate intervention, this can be reduced to as low as 1% (Turner et al., 1989). Consequently, an aggressive therapeutic approach should be adopted. Chlordiazepoxide is an effective means of suppressing the rebound hyperexcitation (tremor, agitation, insomnia). To avoid toxicity owing to its long half-life, shorter-acting benzodiazepines such as lorazepam or oxazepam should be used for elderly patients or those with active liver disease. During withdrawal, care should be taken to ensure adequate hydration and electrolyte replacement.

Any evidence of gastrointestinal bleeding demands a prompt, thorough investigation to discern its orgin. Coagulation parameters should be assessed such as a prothrombin and partial thromboplastin time, a platelet count, and bleeding time.

Most alcohol-related medical problems should be managed in accordance with the accepted standards of medical practice. Long-term rehabilitative efforts typically demand extensive psychosocial counseling following the acute withdrawal period. To improve their chances of remaining sober after leaving the rehabilitation program, patients should also receive vocational training.

INTRAVENOUS DRUG USE

Assessment

Homeless IVDUs are at extremely high risk for developing a wide array of illnesses. One early study estimates that the mortality rate for an IVDU is approximately 16 times greater than that of the general population in the same age group (Duvall et al., 1963). This, coupled with the IVDU's prevailing disinterest in their own physical well-being, creates an extremely challenging problem for the primary care physician.

In general, most medical problems associated with IVDU can be attributed to one of two basic underlying mechanisms.

- Injection of unidentified substance (contaminants) or of known substances in inappropriate dosages (overdosing)
- Practice of unsterile injection techniques that cause abscesses or may give rise to the transmission of infectious diseases such as AIDS or hepatitis

Clinicians who provide care to IVDUs must be familiar with the natural history and clinical findings in several of different disease states. These conditions are listed in Table 7.3 along with some physical findings and treatment considerations. The primary care practitioner, by aggressively treating these complications, can prevent costly hospitalizations, and significantly decrease mortality and morbidity.

Table 7.3 Medical Conditions Associated with Intravenous Drug Use

Condition	Findings, Treatment Considerations
AIDS (common)	Opportunistic infections Weight loss All addicts should receive HIV testing every 6 months
Thrombophlebitis (common)	Tender, superficial veins Doppler examination to assess potency of veins

Table 7.3 (*continued*)

Condition	Findings, Treatment Considerations
Narcotic overdose (common)	Hypotension, decreased respirations Empiric administration of intravenous naloxone hydrochloride (Narcan) (sometimes requires readministration) Maintain airway Be sure to check for comorbid conditions such as head trauma, meningitis
Viral hepatitis (common)	Jaundice, nausea, vomiting, acoric stools, bilirubinuria Patient may be asymptomatic Needs evaluation—blood screening 6 months later to assess for the chronic carrier state
Abscess formation (common)	Often mixed flora (anerobics) with staphylococcal organism Tetanus vaccine, incision, and drainage with iodophor gauze packing Consider antibiotics if evidence of spread is present (cellulitis, lymph adenopathy, fever)
Venous insufficiency (common)	Aggressive therapy for stasis ulcers—impose long-term care on patient to prevent further compromise; elevate legs
Amphetamine psychosis (less common)	Paranoia, manic behavior (may be permanent) Psychiatric referral following medical clearance
Heroin lung (less common)	Dyspnea, "white-out" of lungs on chest radiograph Arterial blood gas to assess need for oxygen, hospitalization
Glomerulonephritis (less common)	Red cell casts in urine, hypertension Check creatinine, blood urea nitrogen
Endocarditis (less common)	Heart murmur, hematuria, conjunctival petechia, splinter hemorrhages

History and Clinical Manifestations

Clinicians should obtain as much information as possible regarding the person's drug usage including drugs being injected, means of administration, and the amount of dosing (including frequency). This information will help the clinician assess mechanisms of injury, risk of certain disease states, and severity of anticipated withdrawal symptoms before entering a detoxification program.

The following information will serve as a point of reference in obtaining a history and trying to characterize a particular patient's addiction profile. Most street drugs sold for intravenous administration are dispensed in "bags" (often condoms or balloons are used) that contain approximately 250 mg of powder or tar. Each bag is melted down in a spoon over an open flame. (Generally, the terms bag and spoon are used interchangeably in reference to quantity.) The liquid is subsequently mixed with tap water and drawn into a syringe, occasionally after first filtering the solution with a ball of cotton. Almost any form of hypodermic can and will be used, but the standard diabetic insulin syringes (selling for $1 to $5 on the street) appear to be used most frequently. When no syringe is available, eyedroppers may be fashioned with a needle and rubber bulb.

According to assays by the Los Angeles police, a typical bag weighs approximately 250 to 300 mg and has approximately a 5% to 7% heroin concentration. The "tar" variety of heroin from Mexico is the most available and usually is of much lower concentrate that the "powder" brought in from Asia called "China white."

Because time for the history is very limited, clinicians should be very direct in asking questions about drug use. Also, when asking questions, it helps to use the street slang. Table 7.4 contains a list of drugs used on the skid row of Los Angeles, slang terminology used on the street, signs and symptoms of chronic use, the means of administration, and possible complications.

We ask patients suspected of intravenous drug use how many bags a day they use. The user may consume an average of 1 to 20 bags of heroin each day. The severity of the withdrawal may be estimated according to the approximate consumption profile of the patient. In general, the greater the amount of heroin being consumed on a regular basis, the sooner the onset and greater the severity of withdrawal symptoms. Given the concentration of heroin in Los Angeles, 1 bag a day is considered a mild habit; 8 bags a day, a medium habit;

and anything from 12 to 20 bags a serious habit. In Los Angeles, because the heroin is so diluted, even a 20-bag-a-day habit does not usually have serious implications for withdrawal.

Clinicians should find out as much as possible about the concentration of heroin in their community. As discussed earlier, the police are a good source of this type of information. Junkies also provide reliable information about what is on the streets. Once they trust you, addicts will keep you informed on changes in drug concentrations or new drugs being sold.

The suspected intravenous drug user should be assessed for common signs of drug use. Some indications of long-standing intravenous drug abuse include emaciation and "tracks" (indurated scars over venous injection sites). Often the addict will have extensive tattoo work to obscure the tracks.

Typically, persons who are injecting cocaine or amphetamines, either alone or in conjunction with other substances, tend to have more extensive scarring than persons who are injecting heroin alone. This may be, in part, owing to the intense vasospasm induced by the cocaine or amphetamines.

The patient may also have abscess formation at the site of dirty injections. "Skin popping" or subcutaneous injection of drugs such as heroin or cocaine leads to superficial sores that subsequently form scars. Impetigo, with its characteristic crusting and honey-colored exudate, is rather common among IVDUs. These lesions are highly contagious and warrant oral antibiotics in addition to local cleaning.

Persons who are acutely intoxicated with narcotics (heroin, demerol, morphine, dilaudid) will have pupillary constriction (miosis, "pinpoint pupils"), dizziness, hypotension, and respiratory suppression.

By contrast, the person who injects stimulants such as cocaine or amphetamines exhibits a distinctly different clinical profile. Acute intoxication results in marked pupillary dilation or mydriasis, tachycardia, pronounced hypertension and, often, bruxism, agitation, tremor and paranoid ideation. Findings may vary when drugs such as heroin and cocaine are used together. This is referred to as "speed balling." Initially the patient exhibits stimulant effects from the cocaine, which is gradually replaced by the depressant effects of the narcotics.

Other signs of intravenous drug use result from the toxic effects of the drug itself, infections caused by dirty needles or needle sharing, or toxic effects of contaminants in the injected drugs (see Table 7.3).

Table 7.4 Drugs Frequently Used on Skid Row

Drug	Slang terminology	Sign and Symptoms of acute intoxication	Signs and Symptoms of chronic use	Means of administration	Possible Complications
Alcohol (ethanol)	Booze Short-dog (wine)	Alcohol odor on breath Slurred speech Impaired coordination Lateral nystagmus Injected sclera Tachycardia (rapid heartbeat)	Tremor Spider telangic-tasia Confabulation Palmar erythema	Oral	Withdrawal (seizures, delirium tremens) Cirrhosis Gastrointestinal hemorrhage Pancreatitis Wernicke-Korsakoff's
Heroin (diacetyl morphine)	Smack China white Mud Carga Cheeva Mr. King	Hypertension Myosis (pinpoint pupils) Hypotension Decreased awareness of surroundings Decreased respirations Nausea, vomiting	Tracks Weight-loss Skin-popping scars Abscesses	Snorting Intravenous Smoking	Overdose coma Endocarditis AIDS Hepatitis Skin abscesses

106

Cocaine	Coke Rock Crack Snow	Hyperexcitation Euphoria Mydriasis (dilated pupils) Hypertension	Depression Weight loss Singed facial hair Perforation of nasal septum	Snorting Intravenous Smoking	Respiratory ailments Sinusitis Paranoia Depression Cardiac dysrhythmias Seizures Pneumothorax Self-mutilation Rhabdomyolyses Seizures Psychosis
Phencyclidine piperdine	Angel dust Kools Sherms	Bizarre, agitated behavior Hypertension Low-grade fever Rapid heart rate Vertical and horizontal nystagmus Ether odor on breath Muscular rigidity	Paranoia, psychosis Impaired memory	Smoking Snorting Intravenous Oral	
Amphetamines	Speed Meth Dexies Crystal Ice	Hypertension Rapid heart rate Markedly dilated pupils Agitation	Weight loss Paranoia Tracks	Oral Intravenous Snorting	Seizures Psychosis Vasculitis Cardiac dysrhythmias

Laboratory Assessment

We offer HIV and Venereal Disease Research Laboratory testing to all IVDUs. Some of our patients agree to the tests, whereas others refuse. Generally, IVDUs not in a program are unwilling to have blood drawn, because they hate needles. For IVDUs in a rehabilitation program, we will do a chemistry panel including liver function tests and a complete blood count. Persons with suspected acute heroin lung who come to the clinic with dyspnea should have a chest radiograph, an EKG, and blood gases.

Treatment

Every effort should be made to optimize the amount of counseling and care provided to the IVDU during each clinic visit. Attempts at education should not be too overwhelming, and should be tempered according to the mental status of the patient and his or her level of trust. As these patients become more comfortable with clinic personnel, it becomes more appropriate to expand on concepts of hygiene, disease prevention, and considerations regarding rehabilitation.

Routine consideration should be given to the following topics:

- HIV status, use of condoms, avoidance of needle sharing, and AIDS education
- Tetanus vaccination status
- Tuberculosis screening (PPD, chest radiograph)
- Referral to rehabilitation programs
- Nutrition status including vitamin supplementation
- Access to food, shelter, and clothing

Many conditions such as impetigo and abscesses can usually be treated in the primary care setting; however, any suggestion of systemic involvement (such as ascending lymphangitis, endocarditis, or a fever) demands referral to a hospital setting.

Following discharge from a hospital, the chances that the patient will comply with follow-up visits to the clinic can be improved by offering the person assistance with housing and meals. If the person can be placed in a facility, then "house calls" can be instituted periodically to ensure compliance with medications or other care.

In contrast to the typical daily heroin addict, occasionally heroin is used on an intermittent basis (known as "chipping"). In this situation, the person never actually develops a significant degree of tolerance or addiction. They are subject to overdosing only when there is an abrupt change in the purity of the heroin used.

In this situation, the primary clinician can assist the patient to "detox" on his or her own. The primary care clinician often encounters persons wishing to withdraw from narcotics but has no place to refer them because of the current lack of funding for drug rehabilitation programs. Unlike alcohol and barbiturate withdrawal, narcotic withdrawal is seldom life threatening. Withdrawal from heroin produces symptoms similar to a bad flu. Withdrawal may be viewed as a rebound phenomenon with essentially the opposite manifestation of acute narcotic intoxication. The patient will exhibit agitation, diaphoresis, abdominal cramping, with occasional vomiting and diarrhea. Peripheral vasoconstriction will induce the classic "cold turkey" appearance of the skin. The withdrawal symptomatology tends to peak in intensity between 2 to 4 days with a gradual tapering off thereafter. Mild physiological disturbances may persist for weeks to months afterward; however, most overt symptoms resolve within 1 to 2 weeks following the last dose of narcotics. The foremost concern in the medical management of heroin withdrawal is to avoid dehydration. The combination of protracted vomiting, diarrhea, and diaphoresis may create a rapid imbalance of fluid and electrolytes requiring hospitalization. The remainder of therapy is directed toward symptomatic relief of various aspects of the withdrawal process. Several therapeutic regimens are in use today (listed in Table 7.5) and should be adjusted to meet the specific needs of the individual patient.

Cocaine Abuse

Assessment

In recent years, cocaine use has become a national epidemic. It is particularly common among homeless persons in the skid row district of large cities. Estimates suggest that more than 20 million Americans have tried cocaine, and about 5 million Americans use it on a daily basis.

Statistics regarding its consumption among the homeless are more difficult to come by. A recent survey at the Weingart Medical Clinic in the skid row district of downtown Los Angeles found that approx-

Table 7.5 Suggested Therapeutic Regimens for Narcotic Withdrawal

General measures:
Ensure adequate hydration
Frequent monitoring of vital signs
Frequent reassurance, encouragement

Specific needs:	*Indication for use:*
Methocarbamol (500 mg every 6 hours)	Muscle cramps, fasiculations
Liquid antacids (30ml every 6 hours)	Dyspepsia, excess acid production (may exacerbate diarrhea)
Acetaminophen (700 mg every 6 hours)	Myalgias, arthralgias
Clonidine (0.1 mg orally twice a day)	Rebound hyperexcitation (watch for hypotension)
Chlorpromazine hydrochloride (Thorazine)[a] (50 mg every day)	Insomnia, rebound phenomena, agitation (watch for extrapyramidal symptoms)
Hydroxyzine pamoate (Vistaril)[a] (50 mg twice a day)	Agitation, rebound phenomenon
Promazine hydrochloride (Sparine)[a] (50 mg intramuscularly every 6 hours)	Agitation, rebound phnomenon
Kaolin (Kaopectate) (30 ml three times a day)	Diarrhea

[a]Only one of the items for agitation should be used at a time.

imately 75% of all persons enrolling in drug and alcohol rehabilitation programs cite cocaine abuse as their primary problem.

Cocaine is used predominantly in the powder form (which can be "snorted" through the nose or dissolved in tap water and injected) or in the crystalline form derived from ether distillation. Crystalline cocaine is known as "crack" because when it is smoked in a glass pipe, a characteristic popping or cracking sound occurs.

Cocaine has an extremely short half-life and is highly addictive, both physically and psychologically. These characteristics tend to create a life-style for the cocaine abuser in which he or she is habitually "chained to the pipe." Use of cocaine causes a depletion of neurotransmitters and results in profound depression of the central nervous system. In the immediate situation, the only way the user can avoid the "crash" is by ingesting more and more cocaine.

History and Clinical Manifestations

Obtaining an accurate history from a cocaine addict is at times especially difficult because they often deny their addiction. Clinicians should look for certain behavior patterns that may suggest a cocaine habit including habitually either "losing" their welfare checks or having them stolen within a day or two of the date issued. Cocaine abuse should also be suspected when a patient desperately solicits cash, is willing to accept almost any sum, and asks almost immediately for more.

Clinicians should ascertain an addiction profile including the length of time a patient has been using cocaine, the amount of his or her daily consumption, and the route of administration. Whether a patient snorts, smokes, or injects cocaine will help define what type of health problems to anticipate. Finally, clinicians should ask about family or social ties as well as the specific reasons why the patient began using cocaine as this information is important in determining rehabilitation strategies.

Cocaine exerts its toxic effects in a variety of mechanisms and results in a wide array of problems. Users are frequently afflicted with sinusitis, upper-respiratory ailments, restrictive airway diseases, and perforation of the nasal septum. The deep inhalation and increased intrathoracic pressure can result in a pneumothorax or a pneumomediastinum. The latter exhibits a typical crunching sound on cardiac ausculation, known as "Hammond's crunch."

Prolonged usage of cocaine results in marked weight loss, profound depression, paranoid ideation, and insomnia. Cocaine is also capable of inducing myocardial ischemia and infarction in persons without any prior evidence of compromised coronary perfusion. Confirmation of suspected cocaine use can be made by testing the urine for its principal metabolite (benzoylecgonine), which will persist in detectable levels for 2 to 3 days following its ingestion.

Laboratory Assessment

Unlike the liver disease or macrocytic anemia characteristic of alcohol abuse, there are few known laboratory abnormalities that specifically suggest a history of cocaine abuse. Thus, laboratory tests should be limited to the investigation of specific clinical problems. For example, creatine phosphokinase isoenzymes would be indicated in assessing the possibilities of myocardial infarction in a cocaine user with chest pain.

Treatment

Because the cocaine addict's first priority is obtaining and consuming more cocaine, the patient will usually present to a medical facility only when an acute health problem requires attention. Therefore, as with the alcoholic or IVDU, every effort should be made to provide cocaine addicts with comprehensive care at each visit.

Several aspects peculiar to cocaine require special consideration. Because of neurotransmitter depletion, vitamin supplements become an important aspect of routine primary care for the cocaine addict. Patients should be given a supply of multivitamins, and tryptophan (50 to 100 mg at bed time).

Symptomatic treatment should be administered as indicated for any of the illnesses associated with cocaine abuse. Patients with septal perforation of the nasal mucosa will require ear, nose, and throat referral for definitive therapy.

Cerebrovascular accidents and cardiac ischemia or dysrhythmias in otherwise healthy individuals have been documented in persons using cocaine. Anyone presenting with chest pain and a history of recent cocaine ingestion warrants a chest radiograph and EKG in addition to a physical examination, regardless of age or the existence of other risk factors.

Sexual favors are often exchanged in the skid row area to obtain more cocaine. Consequently, persons trading sex for cocaine (known as "strawberries") are at increased risk for developing STDs such as AIDS. Thus, persons using cocaine should be counseled about STDs and treated comprehensively for any suspected venereal diseases. An ample supply of condoms should be offered at each clinic visit.

An acute toxic overdose of cocaine can be managed with intravenous propanolol to control sympathomimetic effects of cocaine. Standard therapy should be instituted for controlling hypertension. Intravenous valium is appropriate for control of seizure activity. The abrupt onset of a headache of severe intensity may be a reflection of intracranial or subarachnoid hemorrhage and should be assessed with a computed axial tomographic scan.

The depression induced from cocaine withdrawal can be severe in intensity and may require psychiatric assistance. Somnolence and hyperphagia are also exhibited during the withdrawal state. The goal of medical intervention must be access into a rehabilitation program to treat the patient's addiction. Clinicians should be aware of existing programs in their vicinity, and any regulations or requirements for admission into the program. To reduce the craving for more cocaine during withdrawal, several agents have proved to have some effect, including tricyclic antidepressants, lithium, and vitamin supplementations. Ultimately, however, successful rehabilitation from cocaine requires a multidisciplinary approach including medical, psychiatric, and social counseling.

CONCLUSION

The homeless population frequently resorts to alcohol and drug abuse to try and escape the grim circumstances of their lives. This chapter helps to illustrate how substance abuse can impose further hardships on people who are already in a seemingly hopeless predicament. It is, therefore, all the more important for homeless health care providers to assume a compassionate approach when caring for this population. It is hoped that this chapter assists readers to understand the special medical needs of the homeless substance abuser and, in doing so, leads to improved treatment and rehabilitation programs.

REFERENCES

Brickner P, Scharer, L. K., Conanan B., et al. (Eds.) (1985). *Health care of homeless people*. New York: Springer.

Turner, et al. (1989). Alcohol withdrawal syndromes. *Journal of General Internal Medicine*, 4, 436.

Wright, J. D., Knight, Weber, E., Burdin, Lam, J. et al., (1987). Ailments and alcohol: Health status among the drinking homeless. *Alcohol Health and Research World*.

Human Immunodeficiency Virus and Homeless Persons

8

Robin K. Avery, James J. O'Connell

CHAPTER HIGHLIGHTS

- In recent years, the number of homeless individuals infected with HIV has grown alarmingly.
- Homeless health care programs should monitor for early signs of HIV-related illness, institute prompt treatment, and enroll homeless persons in both standard and experimental therapeutic protocols.
- Despite the pressure to test all homeless persons for HIV infection, health care providers should avoid routine AIDS testing. HIV testing should only be offered in a personal setting with continuity of follow-up, and careful attention to consent and counseling.
- AIDS education of shelter guests and staff should include an emphasis on safe sex, safe needle use, and sensible shelter safety guidelines.
- The complex symptomatology of AIDS is presented from constitutional symptoms to organ-specific signs and symptoms of the skin, eyes, oropharynx, lymph nodes, lungs, heart, intestine, kidneys, genitourinary tract, blood, and neurological systems.
- Management of HIV-related illness includes zidovudine (AZT) and PCP prophylaxis made available at a local community health center or homeless shelter.
- A multidisciplinary team approach to the treatment of AIDS can greatly improve the quality of life for homeless AIDS patients.

INTRODUCTION

With each year of the AIDS epidemic, the number of homeless individuals infected with HIV has grown alarmingly. The Robert Wood Johnson Foundation's National Health Care for the Homeless Program, begun in 19 cities in March 1985, reported only 32 cases of AIDS through March 1987. In Boston, only one person had been diagnosed with AIDS while living in the shelters or on the streets in the spring of 1985. By the end of 1988, however, the Boston Health Care for the Homeless Program had cared for almost 50 persons with AIDS and several hundred with known HIV seropositivity.

Although the exact number of infected persons remains a matter of debate, HIV-related illness in the homeless population undoubtedly constitutes an unprecedented challenge to the systems that have traditionally provided health care to indigent people. New programs and creative solutions are desperately needed. HIV-seropositive homeless persons are entitled to excellent primary and specialized health care, with full access to all diagnostic and therapeutic developments shown to reduce morbidity and mortality in the general population.

Our experience confirms that it is possible among homeless persons to establish a clinical relationship, monitor for early signs of HIV-related illness, institute prompt treatment, and enroll our patients in both standard and experimental therapeutic protocols.

This chapter presents an approach to the homeless person with HIV-related illness, incorporating issues surrounding HIV testing and counseling, clinical assessment, and organization of care. Our intent is to provide a starting point for groups developing models of care to respond to this overwhelming epidemic.

HUMAN IMMUNODEFICIENCY VIRUS TESTING AND COUNSELING

At the present time, no definitive treatment protocol exists for asymptomatic HIV seropositive persons. HIV testing has therefore become an exceedingly sensitive ethical, legal, and public health issue. As debate continues about the propriety of testing under various circumstances and within various groups, consideration of the special needs of those persons without homes is imperative.

Two of our first three HIV-seropositive patients, on learning of their diagnosis, committed suicide. The following story illustrates the need for special care in HIV testing among the homeless:

> In September 1985, a 38-year-old man with a history of intravenous drug abuse (IVDA) since high school presented distraught because of a positive HIV test that had been drawn while in a detoxification unit for alcohol abuse. No counseling had been provided, the patient had been suffering withdrawal from both alcohol and heroin when told that he "ought to have the test taken" to protect himself and others. The patient saw the positive test result as a death sentence, had no reason to stop his substance abuse, and gave up hope of ever having a home. He attempted to hang himself in his jail cell after an arrest for shoplifting. After a short stay in the intensive care unit of a local hospital, he was transferred to a psychiatric facility for observation. The day after discharge, he left his girlfriend a note apologizing for "the travesty that was my life" and overdosed on heroin.

Our experience strongly suggests that HIV testing has failed to be an effective tool in changing behavior patterns in this particular population. Persons without homes, suffering from powerful addictions to heroin or cocaine, find little reason to give up drugs when told of an imminently fatal disease. Despite innovative programs of education, counseling, drug treatment, and support groups, few if any of our patients with frank AIDS have completely abandoned the use of intravenous drugs, and many have continued to share needles despite thorough knowledge of the virus and its transmission.

HIV testing must therefore be treated with the utmost sensitivity in the homeless population. If behavior modification is the goal, then testing must be accompanied by the availability of a stable living situation such as an apartment or a long-term therapeutic community.

Testing should be done only when an excellent support system is in place, with pretest and posttest counseling, referrals for medical care, addictions services including methadone maintenance programs and therapeutic communities, psychiatric services, and full social services with access to appropriate entitlements such as Supplemental Security Income. Skilled interpreters or bilingual care providers are essential given the variety of cultural attitudes toward AIDS.

Counseling must emphasize modes of HIV transmission, differentiation between HIV seropositivity and clinical AIDS, and an open discussion of high-risk behavior. Patients should understand that although the virus has no cure, primary medical care assists in the early detection and treatment of HIV-related illness.

Recent studies have found that AZT is effective in early AIDS-related complex (ARC) and in asymptomatic individuals with low T4 counts. In addition, the availability of aerosolized pentamidine and other forms of PCP prophylaxis make it beneficial for an asymptomatic person with low T4 counts to be tested. It is extremely important to approach testing with caution and sensitivity, however. Undoubtedly, the new findings mentioned earlier will lead to increased pressure to test early; political pressures may also result from the burgeoning numbers of news headlines about HIV in the homeless population. What must be avoided at all costs is a situation in which homeless persons are tested on a large scale in an impersonal setting, without continuity of follow-up or careful attention to consent and counseling. We believe that the benefits of early testing would be lost to individuals tested in such a "mass production" manner. For any individual, to establish the kind of primary care relationship and network of care needed to maintain compliance with AZT or PCP prophylaxis requires a great deal of pretest intervention. Thus, the recent news, although making early testing more desirable from a medical standpoint, mandates an adequate "safety net" of social services, addiction services, and a primary care relationship.

Project Trust, based at Boston City Hospital and funded by the Massachusetts Department of Public Health, offers anonymous testing services, counseling, referrals, and advocacy for a population composed primarily of IVDUs. Our program refers all homeless persons seeking HIV testing to Project Trust; in turn, homeless persons with positive tests are referred directly to our clinic for primary care, whether ill or asymptomatic. This invaluable network has provided an essential safety net for those persons without homes who suffer from drug addiction and who now must face death.

EDUCATION AND ADVOCACY

Homeless health care providers must play a vital role in the AIDS education of shelter guests and staff. Homeless people often feel alienated from society; the diagnosis of AIDS further stigmatizes persons within the shelter community. Educational programs within shelters can present sensible guidelines to assure the safety of all. Such guidelines should include the use of gloves whenever dealing with guests who are bleeding, provision of disposable razors and toothbrushes, disposal of potentially infectious material in appropriate bags (for soft materials) or impervious containers (for sharp items such as needles and razors), and easy accessibility to masks or mouthguards for performing cardiopulmonary resuscitation. Emphasis should be placed on the fact that AIDS is not transmitted by casual contact, handshakes, hugs, touching, or toilet seats. HIV-seropositive persons do not require separate utensils, towels, laundry facilities, or sleeping quarters. All spills of blood, vomitus, stool, or other bodily fluids should be thoroughly cleaned with a 1:10 dilution of sodium hypochlorite (ordinary household bleach). These cleaning procedures should be used for all guests and in all situations, assuring the safety of both staff and guests while minimizing the potential of discrimination toward particular individuals.

Shelters and soup kitchens should be encouraged to display educational posters and programs in English, Spanish, and other relevant languages. Telephone numbers of AIDS advocacy groups should be posted in prominent positions. Condoms and bleach, with understandable instructions and illustrative pamphlets, should be readily available.

Preventive education is the best tool available to thwart the continued spread of HIV. We cannot overemphasize the importance of an organized and persistent program that teaches safer sex and safe needle use to all guests in shelters, regardless of HIV status.

ASSESSMENT

The clinician faces a complex task when a homeless person is referred for care following a positive test for HIV antibodies. The provider must do the following:

- Attempt to assess the severity of any acute conditions
- Determine the extent of HIV-related disease
- Verify test results and inquire about previous health care
- Assess knowledge of both HIV-related illness and the risk factors for transmission of the virus
- Investigate housing and benefit status
- Watch for any signs of neuropsychiatric problems
- Provide the reassurance and support necessary to establish trust

Although it is impossible to accomplish all of this in an initial encounter, enough time must be allotted to the first visit to assure the person that the provider will continue to address his or her multiple needs.

The difference between clinical AIDS and a positive test must be reviewed. For homeless persons, knowledge of AIDS often consists solely of the painful vision of friends dying in the streets. Emphasis should be placed on the highly individual nature of HIV-related illness. We speak hopefully of people who have continued to live productively after diagnosis, who have managed to quit drugs and help themselves and others to achieve better lives. Finally, therapeutic decisions must be in the control of the individual; the provider's role should be collaborative in assisting the patient to make informed decisions.

Confidentiality must be assured to each homeless person with AIDS. Protection of individual privacy is painstakingly difficult in the very public shelters, and most homeless persons are frightened to reveal symptoms to any providers for fear of stigmatization.

SYMPTOMS

AIDS is a complicated illness involving every organ system.

Constitutional Symptoms

After the basis of the therapeutic relationship has been discussed, clinicians should proceed to more specific questions relating to the person's health. The presence and duration of constitutional symptoms, such as fevers, chills, nightsweats, fatigue, loss of appetite, and weight loss, is of primary importance. Documentation of such symptoms is essential not only for the diagnosis of AIDS but also for determination of eligibility for disability. Patients with symptomatic HIV-related illness qualify for Supplemental Security Income and Medicaid. These entitlement programs assure that medications and specialized care will not be denied, and increase chances for housing and placement in drug treatment facilities. All symptomatic patients should be referred immediately to the local Social Security office.

The differential diagnosis of constitutional symptoms is unfortunately vast, especially in a population with a high incidence of substance abuse. Tuberculosis, endocarditis, and malignancy must be thoroughly investigated before the symptoms are attributed to AIDS or ARC. Weights should be recorded at each visit, and the patient should be asked about sources of food and regularity of meals. Homeless persons may be educated about proper nutrition, but the availability of nutritional diets is rare in the shelters and soup kitchens of most cities. We always prescribe multivitamins for our AIDS and ARC patients; for those who have concomitant problems with alcoholism, thiamine and folate are also prescribed.

Skin

Patients should first be asked about recent rashes. Common dermatological conditions such as seborrheic dermatitis and psoriasis are found with increased frequency in HIV-seropositive persons including those who remain otherwise asymptomatic. Providers must be thoroughly familiar with the violaceous and often subtle lesions of Kaposi's sarcoma, the vesicular eruptions of herpes simplex and herpes zoster (which may be atypical or generalized in immunocompromised persons), and the rash of secondary syphilis. Varieties of HIV-related dermatitis, which may be related to the autoimmune manifestations of the disease, have been identified with increasing frequency. Several of our patients have presented with staphylococcal cellulitis in the setting of HIV dermatitis. Other causes of skin lesions, such as scabies and insect bites, must not be overlooked in the homeless population. Drug eruptions are commonly seen in patients receiving medications such as trimethoprim-sulfamethoxazole (TMP-SMZ).

Skin lesions may be systemic or progressive and require hospital admission for full evaluation. In the shelter setting, potentially infectious lesions such as herpes zoster require appropriate public health measures, which usually means admission to an acute care hospital, a medical respite unit, or any facility where the patient can be isolated while receiving appropriate care.

Most commonly, a patient will present with a dermatitis of unclear etiology but that does not appear to require immediate referral. In such cases, a serological test for syphilis should be drawn, a Tzanck preparation performed for any vesicular lesions, and skin biopsies should be done when indicated.

Established or suspected Kaposi's sarcoma mandates a full evaluation of the extent of the disease. One must examine for cutaneous lesions, enlarged lymph nodes, and hepatosplenomegaly. The work-up should include a chest radiograph and possibly an abdominal computed tomographic or thallium scan to determine the presence of visceral lesions. When applicable, such patients should be referred for endoscopy.

Eyes

Blurry vision, diplopia, blind spots, and unusual lights or objects in the visual field are indications for a baseline ophthalmological examination with dilation. Retinal lesions should be promptly referred to an ophthalmologist for evaluation and follow-up. Cytomegalovirus retinitis has caused blindness in many persons with AIDS, and therapy with dehydroxyphenylglycol (Ganciclovir) is required if hematological parameters permit. Intravenous therapy is initiated in the hospital, followed by maintenance intravenous therapy on a long-term basis, which is usually administered at home. Alternative arrangements must be made for those living in shelters, again illustrating the costly logistics of caring for AIDS patients who have no stable living situation.

OROPHARYNX

The mouth should be carefully examined at each visit. Oral candidiasis, hairy leukoplakia, and herpetic lesions are often associated with HIV; common afflictions such as dental caries and periodontal disease may be more frequent in those with HIV seropositivity. Drug reactions such as the oral and perioral lesions of Stevens-Johnson syndrome may occur with common therapies, especially sulfonamide preparations such as TMP-SMZ.

When oral candidiasis has been identified, the provider must determine whether there is esophageal involvement. Persons with oral thrush must be asked about dysphagia, odynophagia, and retrosternal chest pain. Endoscopy is indicated when such symptoms are present. Clinicians should remember, however, that these symptoms may be due to other types of esophageal pathology (e.g., herpesvirus) and that esophagogastric candidiasis can be present with little or no evidence of oral thrush. Treatment of oral thrush consists of local therapy with clotrimazole troches or nystatin suspension. Esophageal candidiasis requires systemic therapy with ketoconazole.

Lymph Nodes

The examination should include the cervical, supraclavicular, axillary, epitrochlear, and inguinal nodes. Generalized adenopathy may be due to HIV infection or a host of other causes, presenting a diagnostic dilemma to the primary care provider. Tuberculosis, Kaposi's sarcoma, and lymphoma can cause diffuse adenopathy and require specific management and therapy. Therefore, a full assessment of adenopathy is usually necessary, particularly if one or more nodes are larger than others, or if the nodes are enlarging with time. Our protocol includes the following: PPD and controls, rapid plasma reagin, heterophile antibody for Epstein-Barr virus, chest radiograph, GU (genito-urinary), and rectal examinations (with appropriate studies such as an immunofluorescence test for chlamydia when inguinal nodes are present). An abdominal computed tomographic scan is required to evaluate the liver and spleen, as well as to determine the presence of retroperitoneal adenopathy. Other laboratory tests should include a complete blood count with differential and platelets, and chemistries including liver function tests.

If one node is particularly prominent, needle aspiration by an experienced practitioner yields a high likelihood of accurate diagnosis. Recent evidence suggests that differential uptake of thallium and gallium provides a clue to the etiology of lymphadenopathy and a guide to further investigation. Bronchoscopy, bone marrow aspirate and biopsy, and upper-gastrointestinal endoscopy may be needed to supplement the preceding diagnostic procedures.

Pulmonary Complications

One of the most feared complications of advanced HIV infection is pneumonia owing to *Pneumocystis carinii*. Florid *P. carinii* with diffuse pulmonary infiltrates, hypoxia, and rapid progression to respiratory failure, represents the final stage of a long process. Indolent *P. carinii* is characterized by a relative lack of pulmonary signs and symptoms, and, thus, a high degree of suspicion must be maintained from the first encounter with an HIV-seropositive patient. Two homeless men in our clinic suffered respiratory arrests following suspected heroin overdoses. Careful investigation determined that each had taken a routine dose of heroin, but the presence of unrecognized pneumocystis in the setting of heroin-related respiratory depression caused the arrests.

Patients with early *P. carinii* may complain of fevers, general malaise, myalgias, headaches, nightsweats, and loss of appetite. A dry cough may be present, but shortness of breath on exertion and easy fatigability may be the only hints of a pulmonary source of infection. The chest radiograph may be clear or suggest only subtle increases in interstitial markings. If early *P. carinii* is suspected, an arterial blood gas is necessary with attention to the arterial-alveolar gradient. Hypoxia or an elevated arterial-alveolar gradient warrants a diagnostic examination of induced sputum, bronchoscopy with lavage, gallium scan, or other procedures depending on individual circumstances and availability.

For HIV-seropositive homeless persons without active *P. carinii* but with low T-helper cell counts, prophylaxis is indicated. A variety of therapies is available including TMP-SMZ, dapsone, and aerosolized pentamidine. Aerosolized pentamidine has considerable advantages for those living in shelters. Administration is required at 2-week intervals, and is thus preferable to medications that must be given once or twice each day. In addition, pentamidine delivered by nebulizer does not add to the hematological toxicity of other medications such as AZT or dideoxyinocine (DDI). The Fenway Community Health Center in Boston has made this treatment available to homeless people, and efforts are currently underway to begin treatment in several shelter clinics and the Medical Respite Unit.

HIV-infected individuals are more susceptible to bacterial pneumonias, typical and atypical tuberculosis (TB and M—atypical mycobacteria), nonspecific interstitial pneumonitis, and pulmonary involvement of cytomegalovirus and Kaposi's sarcoma. More than one of these conditions frequently coexist. Because of the increased incidence of pneumococcal and *Hemophilus influenzae* pneumonia (as well as infections caused by other polysaccharide-encoated bacteria), administration of pneumococcal vaccine is recommended for all adults and children older than 2 years of age who have positive HIV antibodies.

Each HIV-infected patient should have PPD and controls documented, regardless of symptoms, as prophylaxis may be indicated according to the guidelines. Epidemic tuberculosis has been documented among the homeless populations of many cities including New York and Boston. Although tuberculosis was found primarily in elderly alcoholic men living in a particular Boston shelter from 1983 to 1987, most cases of tuberculosis in the past year have been in homeless persons at high risk for HIV-infection. These persons have also had higher incidences of extrapulmonary tuberculosis including renal and pericardial tuberculosis. Given these public health hazards in the crowded shelters of our major cities, we fear for the safety of immunocompromised persons in such conditions. Stable living conditions are imperative, and the discharge of AIDS patients from acute care hospitals to homeless shelters is unacceptable.

Cardiac Problems

Bacterial and fungal endocarditis are prevalent among IVDUs. In addition, persons using cocaine are at higher risk for ischemic heart disease and arrhythmias. AIDS cardiomyopathy is now well documented, and tuberculosis pericarditis is seen with increasing frequency in the homeless population of Boston.

History and physical examination should be supplemented with a chest radiograph and EKG when suspicion of cardiac involvement exists. Hospitalization and broad-spectrum antibiotic coverage pending culture results are indicated when endocarditis is a consideration.

Gastrointestinal Difficulties

Patients should be asked about nausea, vomiting, dysphagia, odynophagia, retrosternal burning, abdominal pain, diarrhea, hematemesis, hematochezia, jaundice, change in color of stools or urine, and rectal pain. If symptoms referable to the esophagus are found, then endoscopy with biopsy can differentiate among candida, herpes, and other causes of esophagitis. Persons with suspected small-bowel disease (unexplained abdominal pain, diarrhea with a nondiagnostic stool examination, evidence of malabsorption) should also be referred for endoscopy with possible duodenal aspirates for parasites, or biopsies for lesions such as lymphoma, typical and atypical mycobacteria, or Kaposi's sarcoma.

Diarrhea should be evaluated with examination of stool for leukocytes, cultures for Salmonella, Shigella, Yersinia, and Campylobacter if indicated, examination for ova and parasites (three samples preferably), and an acid fast stain for Cryptosporidium and atypical mycobacteria. Sigmoidoscopy may be required to diagnose cytomegalovirus colitis, as well as to evaluate rectal pain or lesions noted on routine digital examination of the rectum. The latter can be caused by gonorrhea, herpes, and chlamydia, as well as neoplastic lesions such as the papillomavirus-associated anal carcinoma.

Evidence of liver disease requires liver function tests as well as hepatitis B serology. In the homeless population, alcoholic hepatitis is common, but other etiologies such as non-A, non-B hepatitis, delta hepatitis, disseminated tuberculosis or atypical mycobacteria, and drug reactions must be considered. Abdominal ultrasound or computed tomography will help to rule out parenchymal liver lesions.

HIV-associated biliary disease owing to pathogens such as Cryptosporidium and cytomegalovirus should be considered.

The presence of ascites, whether or not the diagnosis of chronic liver disease has been established, can be due to spontaneous bacterial peritonitis, tuberculous peritonitis, and malignancy.

Renal Abnormalities

HIV-associated renal abnormalities have become increasingly evident, from mild proteinuria to chronic renal failure. Pathologically, the lesion in renal failure is generally focal sclerosis. Use of intravenous drugs, especially heroin, has been associated with nephropathy. Renal function should be monitored regularly, as glomerular filtration rates will dictate medication dosages.

Genitourinary Complications

Thorough examination of the genitalia is necessary for both men and women. STDs must be promptly diagnosed and treated. Malignancy can be detected by testicular examination and cervical Pap smears. Papillomavirus-associated condylomata can be premalignant. Bladder or bowel dysfunction can be due to autonomic neuropathies, infections, or may be early signs of cord compression secondary to malignancy or epidural abscess. A recent homeless patient in our clinic had been seen in several local emergency departments with complaints of low-back pain during a 2-week period. Our nurse practitioner knew that this patient was not a drug user, and persuaded the house staff to admit him for further evaluation. Within 72 hours, he complained of urinary retention and developed lower-extremity paralysis. At surgery he was found to have cord compression secondary to an epidural non-Hodgkin's lymphoma.

Herpetic lesions should be treated with oral acyclovir to minimize the risk of dissemination; however, recent studies have shown the development of resistance to acyclovir by the virus, and new therapies must be developed.

A dramatic increase in the incidence of syphilis has accompanied the AIDS epidemic. All HIV-seropositive persons should have an initial rapid plasma reagin test. When history, physical examination, and subsequent serology suggest any stage of syphilis, recent articles have advocated an aggressive approach based on the findings of accelerated neurosyphilis in some HIV-seropositive individuals treated with traditional regimens. Therefore, a low threshold for performing lumbar puncture should be maintained.

Hematological Abnormalities

A wide spectrum of hematological abnormalities are associated with HIV infection. Providers must be thoroughly familiar with T-cell subsets. Our approach has been to determine T-cell counts early in the evaluation process. T-cell subsets, and the absolute T-helper cell count in particular, assist in the determination of eligibility for AZT, aerosolized pentamidine, and entry into clinical trials of new agents. In addition, T-cell subsets provide information needed to determine medical disability. Whenever possible, T-cell subsets are drawn in the absence of acute infection.

The initial evaluation should include a complete blood count with differential and platelet count. Thrombocytopenia is common and often related to the immune thrombocytopenia of HIV, which may respond to AZT as well as to conventional therapy for ideopathic thrombocytopenic purpura. Anemia is common in this population and may have multiple causes. Screenings for nutritional deficiencies, hemolysis, and gastrointestinal blood loss are necessary. Leukopenia may be due to HIV infection directly, to intercurrent marrow suppression by medications, or to destruction of leukocytes (particulary neutrophils) by autoantibodies. A bone marrow examination may be indicated to rule out malignancy or infection. In atypical mycobacterial infection, granulomas may not be seen, and cultures should be sent whenever a bone marrow is performed.

Therapy with AZT and other antiretrovirals requires close supervision of hematological parameters. Concomitant use of other medications such as TMP-SMZ for *P. carinii* or pyrimethamine and sulfadiazine for toxoplasmosis may result in significant marrow toxicity and should be carefully monitored, particularly for patients living in shelters or on the streets.

Neurological Conditions

HIV can cause a wide spectrum of neurological conditions. Psychiatric illness in the HIV-infected person is a diagnostic and management dilemma. HIV may cause psychosis or affective disorders, or may exacerbate preexisting psychiatric illness. HIV dementia or encephalopathy has been well described, with characteristic early deficits such as poor attention span, memory lapses, and changes in social interactions. In the homeless population, such subtle changes are often overlooked in the setting of substance abuse, chronic mental illness, and the anxiety and sleeplessness that are frequently seen in noisy shelters.

Detailed neuropsychological testing, if available, can assist in the evaluation of cognitive deficits, although this must be done in conjunction with a thorough medical evaluation to exclude infections, structural neurological problems, and metabolic abnormalities.

Shelters are inappropriate for persons with progressive HIV dementia. Our experience suggests that more than one half of our HIV-seropositive patients exhibit some clinical signs of neurological involvement. As the following case study shows, appropriate, supervised facilities for young people with dementia are urgently needed.

A 28-year-old man with a history of remote intravenous drug use was diagnosed with AIDS and central nervous system toxoplasmosis on presentation. He responded to treatment and returned to a local shelter. His behavior became inappropriate, and he left bloodied razor blades in the sinks. Neuropsychiatric evaluation determined mild dementia, although the patient was not felt to be incompetent. Although he was on Supplemental Security Income, Medicaid was unable to cover placement in a nursing home because of his young age, and he returned to the streets. He slept most nights between the glass doors in the entryway to a shelter, where the clinic staff could tend to his basic needs. Unfortunately, he was found dead on a street corner several months later.

A neurological evaluation of the HIV-seropositive person with an acute or subacute problem generally includes a lumbar puncture and a computed tomographic scan of the head. The cerebrospinal fluid (CSF) should be examined for cell count and differential, gram stain, and routine cultures; acid-fast bacilli smear and culture; fungal preparation and culture; cryptococcal antigen; and venereal disease. HIV in the central nervous system can directly cause a mild pleocytosis, elevated CSF protein, and other abnormalities. Cryptococcal meningitis may have a subacute presentation with few meningeal signs. Long-term therapy with amphotericin has been prescribed in the past, but recent studies with the experimental oral medication fluconazole have shown considerable promise.

Neurosyphilis deserves special consideration. Any abnormality noted on CSF examination, regardless of the Venereal Disease Research Laboratory result, merits serious consideration for treatment of neurosyphilis in patients with a previous history or present evidence of clinical syphilis or a positive-serum rapid plasma reagin–fluorescent treponemal antibody test.

Computed tomographic scan with contrast might reveal the ring-enhancing lesions of toxoplasmosis; other possible findings include lymphoma, progressive multifocal leukoencephalopathy, tuberculoma, and cerebral atrophy without focal lesions. More than one condition, for example, toxoplasmosis and lymphoma, may coexist and be difficult to differentiate by computed tomographic scan alone. A brain biopsy is sometimes indicated when a definitive diagnosis is necessary, or when antitoxoplasmosis therapy has failed.

An encephalitis with clouded consciousness and progression to coma can be produced by herpes simplex, cytomegalovirus, varicella zoster, toxoplasmosis, and HIV (though the latter is generally more indolent). When prescribing medications for the chronic mentally ill homeless person, providers should remember that patients with underlying HIV infection of the CNS may be more sensitive to the side effects of psychoactive medications.

Peripheral neuropathies resulting from HIV, with painful paresthesias and numbness in the extremites, are seen frequently and are very difficult to distinguish from alcoholic neuropathy. HIV-associated conditions of the spinal cord, such as vacuolar myelopathy, may produce progressive debilitation and disability.

Baseline neurological functioning and mental status should be documented during the initial evaluation of the HIV-seropositive patient. Detailed cranial nerve examination should be done at each visit. History of substance abuse or previous psychiatric illness should be noted. This initial documentation is exceedingly important with homeless persons, as subtle changes in behavior may herald significant disease. Shelter staff have a unique opportunity to notice changes in behavior, and cooperation between the shelters and the care providers is essential.

MANAGEMENT OF HUMAN IMMUNODEFICIENCY VIRUS–RELATED ILLNESS

Homeless persons with AIDS are entitled to receive state-of-the-art health care. Providers must assure that these persons have access to the best possible treatment, and should provide the information necessary for each person to make informed and considered decisions concerning enrollment in therapeutic protocols.

AZT ZIDOVUDINE

AZT is the only antiretroviral medication currently licensed in the United States for treatment of HIV infection. There are other anti-retrovirals currently undergoing testing that may be available in the near future. Persons eligible for AZT therapy in the past were those with AIDS or ARC with a low total T-helper count (T4 count) of less than 200. Recent evidence indicates that AZT is likely beneficial for individuals with early ARC or asymptomatic persons with low T4 counts, and we are offering it to all persons in these categories. However, Indications for AZT are rapidly changing, and homeless projects should keep abreast of new recomendations from the Centers for Disease Control.

Our approach has been to describe AZT to eligible individuals, discussing the positive results of the initial AZT study, which appeared in the *New England Journal of Medicine* in September 1987 (Fischel et al., 1988). This study indicated that, of a population with AIDS or advanced ARC, the group that received AZT had fewer deaths and fewer serious infections. Also, later evidence from these study groups found that some of the neurological consequences of HIV infection may be ameliorated by long-term AZT therapy. We also emphasize that AZT has its disadvantages. It must be taken every 4 hours around the clock, and requires a commitment by the person to close medical follow-up and frequent blood drawing.

These requirements present considerable challenges to persons without homes. Venous access in persons with long histories of intravenous drug use is difficult, and blood drawing can be an ordeal for both patient and provider. Compliance with the every-4-hour regimen is very difficult when wandering the streets during the day hours and sleeping in large dormitory-style shelters at night. Special timers and shelter staff committed to waking certain individuals for the night doses have helped many of our patients follow the AZT regime. It is hoped that new drugs with an easier-to-follow regimen will soon be available. We are currently enrolling several homeless persons in the dideoxyinocine trial, in which the medication is given once a day.

Eligible persons who agree to take AZT receive blood work (complete blood count with differential and platelet count, chemistries with liver function tests) as often as every week during the first months of therapy. The full dose of AZT in use up until recently was 200 mg (two 100-mg tablets) every 4 hours; recent evidence suggests that a dose of 100 mg taken every 4 hours is equally effective and less toxic than the previous dose. If isolated anemia is a problem, AZT therapy has been successfully continued with intermittent transfusions. Of clinical importance to the shelter clinics, acetaminophen appears to increase AZT toxicity and should not be given to persons on this medication.

AZT costs more than $7,000 per year per patient. All of our patients with AIDS or ARC receive Medicaid, which currently pays the entire cost of the drug. Medications are frequently lost, stolen, or sold in the shelters and on the streets (AZT has a high value on the black market), however, and replacement can be prohibitively expensive. In addition, the toxicities of AZT and the newer experimental drugs are considerable, and unmonitored consumption on the streets can be life threatening. Therefore, our policy has been to have medications held in the shelter clinics whenever possible, dispensing periodic supplies according to the needs and wishes of the individual.

Phencyclidine Piperdine Prophylaxis

All persons with AIDS or advanced ARC are candidates for prophylaxis against PCP. A good summary of the different modalities can be found in the *Medical Letter* of October 7, 1988. As mentioned previously, aerosolized pentamidine prophylaxis is proving to be an excellent therapy for several homeless individuals. Treatment should be made available at a local community health center as well as homeless shelters.

COORDINATION OF CARE: PRIMARY CARE MODEL

Providers must maximize use of local and national resources to create programs that address the unique needs of the HIV-infected homeless population. The nature of the illness mandates a multidisciplinary team approach to provide primary and specialty care with consistent follow-up and full access to services and benefits that improve the quality of life after diagnosis.

The following story illustrates the network of care that has developed in the Boston area and highlights the strengths as well as the shortcomings of our health care system:

> A 40-year-old black man was admitted to a Boston hospital for elective knee surgery. Oral thrush was noted incidentally by the anesthesiologist during preoperative evaluation. The surgery was

canceled, an HIV test drawn, and the patient was discharged to the shelter. The following morning he went to Project Trust, and an alert staff member brought the patient to our Homeless Clinic at Boston City Hospital. The thrush was treated. The patient resisted initial attempts to establish a primary care relationship, however, and ignored symptoms of shortness of breath, fatigue, and fevers for several weeks. Finally, one of us saw the patient in the AIDS Clinic at Boston City Hospital and admitted him for uneventful treatment of *P. carinii.*

Our team worked closely with the house staff and social workers to arrange an admission to the Medical Respite Unit, a 25-bed facility managed by the Boston Health Care for the Homeless Program in the Lemuel Shattuck Hospital Shelter, where oral Trimethoprim sulfamethoxazole (TMP-SMX) (Bactrim) therapy was continued, and the patient was begun on AZT without difficulty. This respite unit, one of two in the country, is supervised by a physician and nurse practitioner, and offers intermediate care to homeless persons who are too ill or infirm to be walking the streets, but who do not require acute care hospitalization. This man was able to have his medication supervised every 4 hours, receive physical therapy and nutrition counseling, and enroll in an on-site drug and alcoholism treatment program. The project social worker assisted him with entitlement and housing applications. After several weeks, the patient returned to his original shelter. He has formed strong relationships with the nurses in the shelter clinic, who continue to monitor his AZT and to watch for new symptoms. In addition, he is examined each week in the AIDS Clinic, where he also attends a support group and meets with his advocate from the AIDS Action Committee. He remains stable medically, and receives aerosolized pentamidine every other week at the Fenway Community Health Center. After an adverse reaction to AZT, he is now under consideration for the Phase I trial of DDI. All who have cared for this man have been impressed by his extraordinary good humor and warm, unassuming nature.

CONCLUSION

Excellence and consistency in the care of persons with AIDS who have no permanent homes requires an extensive network of services. Each city must respond to this crisis by using existing facilities, while creating new programs and alternatives. The daunting dimensions of this epidemic mandate an organized and collaborative response by society and the health care system.

REFERENCES

Centers for Disease Control. (1987). Revision of the CDC surveillance case definition for acquired immunodeficiency syndrome. *MMWR, 36:* 1S, 3S–15S.

Centers for Disease Control (1985). Summary: recommendations for preventing transmission of infection with human T-lymphotropic virus type III/lymphadenopathy-associated virus in the workplace. *MMWR, 34(45):* 681–689.

Fischl, M. A., et al. (1988). Safety and efficacy of sulfamethoxazole and trimethoprim chemoprophylaxis for Pneumocystis carinii pneumonia in AIDS. *Journal of the American Medical Association, 259,* 1185.

Fischl MA, Richman DD, Grieco MH, Gottlieb MS, Volberding PA, Laskin OL, et al. (1987). The efficacy of azidothymidine (AZT) in the treatment of patients with AIDS and AIDS-related complex: a double-blind, placebo-controlled trial. *New England Journal of Medicine, 317(4):* 192.

Friedland, GH, Saltzman BR, Rogers MF, Kahl PA, Lesser ML, Mayers MM, et al. (1986). Lack of transmission of HTLV III/LAV infection to household contacts of patients with AIDS or AIDS-related complex with oral candidiasis. *New England Journal of Medicine, 314(6):* 344–349.

Freidland GH, & Klein RS. (1987). Transmission of the human immunodeficiency virus: an updated review. *New England Journal of Medicine, 317(18):* 1125–1135.

Libman H, Witzburg RA, (Eds.) (1990). Clinical Manual for Care of the Adult Patient with HIV Infection. Department of Medicine, Boston City Hospital.

Reitmeijer CA, Krebs JW, Feorino PM, Judson FN. (1988). Condoms as physical and chemical barriers against human immunodeficiency virus. *Journal of the American Medical Association,* 259(12): 1851–1853.

Sande MA, Volberding PA, Eds. (1988). The Medical management of AIDS. Philadelphia: WB Saunders Co.

Volberding PA, Lagakos SW, Koch MA, Pettinelli C, Meyers MW, Booth DK, et al. (1990). Zidovudine in asymptomatic human immunodeficiency virus infection: a controlled trial in persons with fewer than 500 CD4-positive cells per cubic millimeter. *New England Journal of Medicine, 322(14):* 941–949.

Weinberg DS, Murray HW. (1987). Coping with AIDS: the special problems of New York City. *New England Journal of Medicine 317(23):* 1469–1472.

Winkelstein W, Lyman DM, Padian N, Grant R, Samuel M, Wiley JA, et al. (1987). Sexual practices and risk of infection by the hyman immunodeficiency virus: The San Francisco Men's Health Study. *Journal of the American Medical Association,* 257(3): 321–325.

Trauma and Victimization

9

Susan Fleischman

CHAPTER HIGHLIGHTS

- Trauma and accidents are the leading causes of illness, disability, and death among the homeless.
- The homeless life-style and barriers to medical care result in delayed treatment of traumatic injuries and more frequent complications such as serious infections, permanent disfigurement, disability, or even death.
- Adequate care for homeless trauma patients requires appropriate triage and medical intervention at the local clinic or emergency department.
- A comprehensive evaluation of homeless trauma victims includes a social and medical history to assess potential barriers to adequate treatment and recovery.
- Daily, close follow-up of trauma patients is crucial to prevent complications; placement in an environment that allows for proper healing and recovery will dramatically improve the outcome for traumatic injuries.
- Lack of a safe shelter, and alcohol and drug abuse make homeless women especially vulnerable to sexual assault.
- Homeless rape victims should be tested for STDs (including AIDS) and treated as STD contacts.
- Essential elements of care for homeless rape victims include crisis counseling, referral to appropriate long-term counseling and legal aid, social services, and emergency safe housing.

INTRODUCTION

Trauma and accidents are the leading causes of illness, disability, and death among the homeless. Without adequate housing, the homeless population is extremely vulnerable to both accidents and violent crime. Mental illness, and drug and alcohol abuse add to this vulnerability.

A 3-year study of 6,000 homeless men in Stockholm found that 20% of 327 deaths during the study period were the result of trauma (Alstrom, Lindlius, & Salum, 1975). Major trauma accounted for one quarter of all admissions of homeless patients to San Francisco General Hospital in 1983 (Kelly, 1985).

In a recent survey of the homeless in Los Angeles, 40% reported that they were victims of an accident or of an acute illness during the past 2 months (Ropers and Boyer, 1987). Broken bones accounted for 31%, and lacerations were 26% of all accidents (Ropers and et al., 1987). At San Francisco General, lacerations were the most frequent result of trauma followed by fractures and contusions (Kelly, 1985).

The homeless also have a high incidence of repeat trauma and hospitalization. Forty-seven percent of the homeless admitted to San Francisco General for major trauma had prior or subsequent hospitalizations at the hospital, and more than one half had been hospitalized for a previous episode of major trauma (Kelly, 1985).

The same factors that cause increased trauma in the homeless are probably responsible for the increased incidence of sexual assault. Lack of safe shelter makes homeless women extremely vulnerable to rape. As with trauma in general, alcohol and drug abuse often add to this vulnerability. In a review of charts at San Francisco General, Kelly (1985) found that although the homeless constitute less than 0.4% of the San Francisco population, 9% of adult victims of sexual assault were homeless. The usual underreporting of rape is compounded for the homeless by the difficulties and barriers faced when seeking medical care. Thus, the incidence of sexual assault may be even higher. The incidence of repeat sexual assault is also high; 12% of the homeless victims of sexual assault had been treated previously for one or more sexual assaults (Kelly, 1985).

NATURAL HISTORY OF THE DISEASES

Homelessness not only increases the risk for trauma and victimization, but also affects outcome once the trauma has occurred. Underlying, untreated chronic illness and malnutrition may complicate treatment and healing of traumatic injuries. At the time of discharge after major trauma, the patient may have wounds that require complex daily care regimens, casts or splints, or prohibitions regarding weight bearing. The likelihood is quite low that wounds will receive appropriate care, that casts will stay in place, and that orthopedic recommendations will be followed. The homeless life-style itself, which requires miles of walking each day to find food and nightly shelter, makes bed rest or leg elevation difficult or impossible, and further complicates wound healing after discharge. As a result, wounds often dehisce and become infected; and fractures often heal poorly, leading to lifetime disability. Unfortunately, problems of follow-up care are rarely considered by the hospital personnel when making a discharge plan for a homeless patient after major trauma. Extended hospitalizations for homeless patients are not encouraged in this era of shortened hospitalizations.

Outcomes after minor trauma are also affected by homelessness. Treatment for non–life-threatening illness may not be a high priority to those struggling for food and shelter. Drug and alcohol use, as well as mental illness, may impair judgment and delay seeking medical care. Finally, extremely long waits at crowded emergency departments discourage homeless patients from seeking care for minor trauma. Wound dehiscence, infection, and inappropriate fracture healing are common after minor trauma is treated in an emergency department with no follow-up. Lack of money for prescriptions, lack of dressing change materials, and lack of appropriate, early follow-up also contribute to poor outcomes for homeless trauma patients.

ASSESSMENT

Homeless trauma victims often first seek care at community clinics, regardless of the severity of the injury. Clinics must be staffed to do emergency triage during all operating hours. Clinic staff may be required to make immediate assessment and initiate life-support measures while awaiting paramedic response.

Minor trauma can often be appropriately handled without referral to a local emergency department, although this will depend on in-clinic capabilities. New lacerations should be examined on an urgent basis so that they may be sutured for primary closure. Delays of more than 24 hours before examining new lacerations may cause wounds to become too old for safe suture placement, leading to chronic wound infections and disability.

Minor trauma, not requiring trauma center care, is probably *better* cared for at a community clinic that is sensitive to the life-style and needs of homeless persons. Because these injuries are not life threatening, they are of low priority in emergency departments. Many homeless clients who seek care at emergency departments are never actually seen because they are unable or unwilling to wait. Moreover, clinics can give more comprehensive health care and more social service intervention than emergency departments. Often, the presenting minor complaint for which the patient seeks care is insignificant compared with other medical and mental health problems that can be found during a comprehensive history and examination. The busy emergency department will not perform comprehensive histories or examinations.

Triage of rape victims will depend on the capabilities of the clinic and how long ago the rape occurred. If legal collection of evidence can be performed on-site, it should be done as soon as possible. Otherwise, the victim should be transported to the appropriate agency for evidence collection. Rape victims who first seek care days or weeks after the rape should be seen in the clinic the same day they present.

For all trauma patients, in addition to taking the routine history regarding the trauma, the clinician should obtain a complete social history including mental health status, alcohol and drug use, and the patient's current housing situation. Whether a trauma patient stays in a shelter, on the street, or in SRO is particularly important for decisions regarding treatment and follow-up. With appropriate home visits, an injury that might heal in a patient living in an SRO may require hospitalization in a mentally disabled individual who is wandering the streets.

Past medical history and review of systems should be done regardless of the chief complaint. Often a more serious but neglected problem may become apparent. Coexisting illnesses often not mentioned by clients at the time of presentation for minor trauma include hypertension, diabetes, cirrhosis, and tuberculosis. Coexisting illness or medication use will affect the patient's treatment and follow-up.

The physical examination should be as comprehensive as possible including an assessment of overall health status and personal hygiene. Poor general health status and hygiene as well as the existence of comorbid conditions will increase the risk of infection, delay recovery time, and increase the chance of permanent disability.

The laboratory assessment should include a hematocrit if significant blood loss is suspected and radiographs if a fracture is suspected. Radiographs should be read immediately, so that if there is a fracture present, the patient can be referred for immediate reduction and stabilization.

TREATMENT

Major Trauma

The clinic staff should be trained in basic life-support measures. Emergency equipment that should be available includes an ambu-bag, oxygen, intravenous needles and fluids, and a crash cart with emergency medications and a defibrillator. The clinic should establish a good relationship with the local paramedics to ensure a rapid and appropriate response. Relationships with local emergency departments are also critical; working with the referral system to identify patients as homeless will help the emergency department provide appropriate evaluation and treatment, and may influence its decision to hospitalize the patient.

Minor Trauma

Treatment for minor trauma often depends on the age of the injury, especially when dealing with lacerations. The homeless commonly present with wounds and lacerations that occurred more than 24 hours before treatment is sought.

New lacerations should be immediately cleansed, debrided, and sutured if appropriate. If suturing is not done on-site, the patient should be referred to the nearest emergency department. Old wounds should be aggressively cleansed and debrided. Appropriate dressing should be well secured for the wear and tear that will occur before the first follow-up visit.

Clinicians should pay special attention to the patient's tetanus status. Immunization histories are often unreliable. Patients should be given tetanus toxoid, unless the patient can clearly recall a recent tetanus immunization. Tetanus immune globulin should be given to previously nonimmunized individuals and to patients with dirty wounds for which immunization status is unclear. Many homeless trauma victims are aware of tetanus immunization during recent emergency department visits for previous trauma incidents.

If wounds are infected, antibiotics should be given. Prophylactic antibiotic use is indicated in high-risk wounds such as bites, especially human, and old, dirty wounds (see chapter 10 by Usatine on dermatological problems). It is less clear whether prophylactic antibiotics are indicated for patients with underlying illnesses such as diabetes or malnutrition, or for those who simply have poor personal hygiene.

The homeless are often discharged from emergency departments with prescriptions for antibiotics or medical supplies that are never filled. Therefore, before discharge, sufficient wound dressing supplies and medications to last until the first follow-up visit should be given to the patient. These include all necessary supplies required for wound care (i.e., iodine, peroxide, gauze, tape). Appropriate support devices such as ace wraps, splints, and crutches should also be supplied.

Rape

Appropriate treatment of rape victims begins with correct legal collection of evidence. Simultaneously, cultures for gonorrhea and chlamydia should be obtained. Victims should be empirically treated as STD contacts rather than awaiting culture results. To prevent conception, two tablets of norgestrel (Ovral) at the time of examination and two tablets 12 hours later should be given if the rape occurred less than 72 hours before the examination. HIV baseline testing and follow-up testing at 3 months, baseline syphilis serologies, and baseline hepatitis B serologies and repeat serologies in 8 to 12 weeks should also be offered. On-site crisis counseling at the time of the initial visit is optimal, as well as referral to appropriate long-term counseling and legal aid. A careful social history is critical for obtaining nonmedical help for homeless rape victims. Unfortunately, rape victims may have no alternative but to return to the same area where they were raped, or return to an abusive relationship, on which they are dependent. Social services and emergency, safe housing should be offered to all rape victims.

AFTERCARE AND FOLLOW-UP

The most difficult part of treating trauma in the homeless population begins after discharge from the hospital, emergency department, or clinic. Standard protocols for cast checks and wound checks must be altered to take into account the high rate of complications owing to the homeless life-style. For major trauma patients, discharge from an acute care hospital to the street without proper follow-up can cause serious complications and permanent disability. Hospital social workers deal mainly with a domiciled population. If they do not regularly deal with homeless persons and homeless service agencies, the hospital may not provide appropriate discharge planning. A clinic social worker, who is in touch with the homeless agency network, is in a better position to smooth the transition from hospital to street. This transition sometimes requires placement in a board-and-care facility, if available, or at least the provision of temporary respite beds either in local shelters or through hotel voucher programs. Ideally, a clinic-based social worker or case manager will follow the patient from an initial emergency department referral and hospitalization; be aware of eminent discharges; and, working with hospital social workers and providers, assist in discharge planning.

Medical follow-up after discharge should be offered at local clinics. Hospital clinics are often unable to accommodate the homeless because they have tight appointment schedules, limited hours, and no system for rescheduling broken appointments or follow-up of "no shows." If hospital medical records are unavailable, or there is no clear understanding of what occurred during the hospital stay, however, it is difficult for the clinic practitioners to determine what follow-up care is needed. A good relationship with local hospitals facilitates proper referrals and makes it easier to obtain needed medical records. If a referral back to the hospital-based clinics is necessary, clinic staff can act as advocates for the patient in obtaining necessary appointments, aiding with transportation, and so forth.

Victims of minor trauma may also do poorly after discharge from emergency departments or clinics. Injuries to the lower extremities often require elevation of the legs or even nonweight bearing. This is impossible for most homeless patients, even those in shelters. Likewise, appropriate wound care is difficult for those living on the street. Finding respite beds through social service networking may be as important as wound cleansing and antibiotics. Referral for temporary disability entitlements can be done simultaneously. Referral to a detoxification program may be necessary for the alcohol or drug user who will not be able to take appropriate care of an injury.

Because of the high rate of complications, initial follow-up should be performed daily for wound checks and dressing changes. This is

best done at local clinics, and at outreach sites such as food lines and
SROs. Just enough antibiotics and dressing change materials should
be given at each visit to last until the next dressing change or wound
check.

The charts of patients who fail to appear for a follow-up appointment should be reviewed on a daily basis. Case managers or providers should undertake an active search to find patients who have failed
appointments and who need to be seen. This search may require
extensive networking with social service agencies and public health
nurses. Although searching for no-show patients is time-consuming
and often frustrating, finding patients who have not come in for
follow-up can prevent permanent complications and disability.

CONCLUSION

Homelessness itself is a risk factor for trauma and victimization.
Once traumatized, the homeless have a worse outcome with increased hospitalizations and more permanent disability. Adequate
care requires not only appropriate triage and medical intervention at
the local clinic or emergency department, but also social service
intervention to get the homeless patient off the street and into an
environment that will allow for proper healing and recovery. The
dispensing of appropriate antibiotics and wound care supplies is also
important. Daily close follow-up and the pursuit of patients who fail
to keep appointments will reduce long-term complications. Caring
for the homeless who present with minor trauma presents a challenging opportunity to provide comprehensive health care to a high-risk
population.

REFERENCES

Alstrom, Lindlius, C. H., & Salum, I. (1975). Mortality among homeless
    men. *British Journal of Addiction, 70,* 245–252.
Brickner, B. W., Scharer, L. K., Conanan., B., et al. *Health care of homeless
    people.* New York: Springer.
Olin, J. S. (1966). "Skid row" syndrome: A medical profile of the chronic
    drunkeness offender. *Canadian Medical Association Journal, 95,* 204–
    214.
Ropers, R. H. and Boyer, R. (1987, Spring). Homeless as a health risk.
    Alcohol Health and Research World, 11, 38–41.

Skin Diseases of the Homeless

Richard Usatine

10

CHAPTER HIGHLIGHTS

- The homeless are at high risk for developing skin problems because of exposure to the elements, unsanitary living conditions and lack of hygiene, overcrowding in shelters, poor nutritional status, alcoholism and drug abuse, and exposure to violence and trauma.
- Dermatological disorders are often the commonest diagnosis among homeless patients seeking primary health services.
- The commonest dermatological diagnoses found in homeless patients are bacterial infections (impetigo, cellulitis, and abscess); lacerations; fungal infections; eczema; and lice and scabies.
- Information on the living conditions of a homeless patient as well as a sexual history provides valuable clues in diagnosing skin conditions commonly found in this population.
- Treatment for dermatological problems in homeless patients is often difficult because of the conditions in which they live. For example, the most important treatment for cellulitis of the leg—elevation—is often impossible for a homeless person to carry out.
- Without treatment for the underlying problems of homelessness, skin problems, such as "wine sores" found on the hands, fingers, arms, trunk, and legs of the a homeless alcoholic, will recur time and again.

INTRODUCTION

The homeless are exposed to many risk factors that contribute to the development of dermatologic diseases, frequently more severer and more extensive than found in the general population. This chapter concentrates on the more common conditions seen among the homeless at the Venice Family Clinic Homeless Health Clinic.

RISK FACTORS

The major risk factors that contribute to the development of skin problems in the homeless include the following:

- Exposure to the elements—sun, rain, wind, and dirt
- Unsanitary conditions and poor hygiene
  Limited access to soap and water.
  Soiled and inadequate clothing
  Sharing of dirty clothing, blankets, sleeping bags, hats, and combs with other homeless persons
  Mental illness that may promote resistance to bathing and changing clothing
- Overcrowding in shelters leading to transmission of lice and scabies, and other contagious skin disorders
- Poor nutritional status leading to poor wound healing
- Alcoholism
- Drug abuse (use of dirty needles causing skin abscesses and cellulitis)
- Exposure to violence and trauma (lacerations, abrasions, burns, etc.)
- Barriers to seeking medical care resulting in delayed treatment of skin problems

GENERAL ASSESSMENT

When a homeless person is complaining of a "rash" or a problem with the skin, the assessment begins as with any other patient, with a good history and physical examination. Because in dermatology "a picture is worth a thousand words," in most cases, the visual inspection of the patient's skin is 90% of the assessment.

The health care provider should be able to characterize the lesions observed in terms of type of lesion (macule, papule, pustule, vesicle, bullae, plaque, ulcer, crust, scale); sites and distribution; duration of lesions; and history of pruritis.

In addition to visual inspection, answers to several questions will help the practitioner diagnose and treat common dermatologic problems. For example, to provide appropriate treatment, the practitioner should ask whether the patient currently lives on the streets or in a shelter; whether they share cramped sleeping quarters, blankets, garments, or combs; if they have been able to bathe and wash their clothing lately; their eating habits; any recent trauma; and problems with alcohol and drug abuse.

A sexual history is essential because many STDs present with skin lesions. This information is therefore needed for adequate diagnosis, treatment, and counseling. Any lesion on the genitalia, in the groin, or perirectal region should alert practitioners to the possibility that they are dealing with a STD.

COMMON SKIN DISORDERS

Dermatologic disorders are the most common diagnoses seen among the homeless seeking primary care at the Venice Family Clinic. The following is a listing of the major categories of dermatologic problems seen among the homeless clinic population at the Venice Family Clinic as a percent of total visits. We discuss each category of conditions from the most to least common.

Bacterial Infections	24.2%
Impetigo	9.6%
Cellulitis	8.0%
Abscess	6.6%
Lacerations	14.5%
Fungal infections	8.2%
Eczema	7.8%
Lice and scabies	7.6%

BACTERIAL INFECTIONS

The largest group of skin disorders seen among the homeless consists of the bacterial skin infections (e.g., impetigo, cellulitis, and abscess).

Impetigo

Impetigo is very common among homeless adults as well as homeless children. Impetigo is defined as "an acute purulent infection which is at first vesicular and later crusted—a very superficial infection of the skin due to group A streptococci and often Staphylococcus aureus, or a mixed infection" (Fitzpatrick et al., 1983).

One variation of typical impetigo is the "wine sore" found on the hands, fingers, arms, trunk, and legs of the homeless alcoholic. These impetiginized lesions are especially seen on the dorsum of the hands and over the knuckles of the fingers (see Figures 10.1 and 10.2) Below the crusts or scabs is a purulent white base. The pathophysiological process probably starts with mild trauma to the area allowing bacteria to enter into the epidermis and dermis. This may happen as the alcoholic sleeps on the ground or is digging through a garbage can or dumpster for food. Occasionally, these sores present in nonalcoholics who collect aluminum cans from garbage for recycling. A lack of cleanliness, poor nutrition, and poor general health cause lesions to fester and become chronic, unless treated adequately.

To treat impetigo, it is important to choose an antibiotic that covers streptococcus and *Staphylococcus aureus*, such as erythromy-

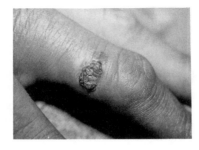

FIGURE 10.1 Impetigo of finger—"wine sore" or echthyma.

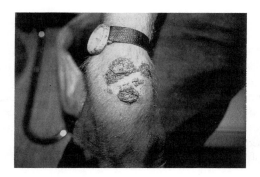

FIGURE 10.2 Impetigo in alcoholic man living on streets.

cin and dicloxacillin. Treatment should be for 10 consecutive days.

The antimicrobial treatment of "wine sores" is the same as impetigo. Treatment should also include the debridement of the overlying scab or crust. Once the scab is removed with forceps or firm rubbing with gauze, the base of the lesion should be cleaned with hydrogen peroxide or betadine. Sterile dressings can then be applied. Topical antibiotics such as bacitracin may also be applied under the dressing. If the lesions are large or numerous, a systemic antibiotic will be beneficial.

Because adequate medical care for many bacterial skin infections requires daily dressing changes, the patient should return daily to the clinic. This is especially important if the patient is not mentally or physically able to perform a dressing change. In some cases, the patient or a patient's friend may be taught to do the dressing change and then given the necessary materials to carry out the wound care outside the clinic. If a patient or partner is unable to care for the impetigo, he or she is given only one day of antibiotics at each visit and encouraged to return daily for treatment. To encourage compliance, follow-up visits should be convenient and clinic waiting time kept to a minimum.

The presence of wine sores is an opportunity to discuss the patient's alcoholism. We explain that his or her sores are related to drinking alcohol and that part of the treatment is to stop drinking. Because these wine sores are so visible, they make it more difficult for the patient to deny the effects of alcohol on the body. Providers should use every opportunity to encourage detoxification and sobriety. When the patient is receptive to treatment, appropriate counseling and referral should be provided.

Cellulitis

Cellulitis is defined as an acute infection of the skin involving the deeper subcutaneous tissues. The most common etiologic agents are group A beta-hemolytic streptococci and *S. aureus*, but other bacteria may be involved (Fitzpatrick et al., 1987). In the homeless, cellulitis is most commonly seen in the extremities, complicating untreated trauma (lacerations or human bites), peripheral vascular disease, and intravenous drug access infections.

One type of cellulitis seen on the legs of homeless patients with peripheral vascular disease is called "mission legs." Mission legs is a term used to describe massive pedal edema from poor venous return, exacerbated by the person sleeping in an upright position (e.g., in a car, on a bench, in a chair, or on the pews of a mission or church). Following a break in the skin in which bacteria are introduced, the chronic venous stasis predisposes the person to cellulitis. In chronic venous stasis, the skin tissues are compromised because of poor oxygenation and impaired circulation. This skin is unable to fight the infection effectively, and the cellulitis spreads easily to involve the whole lower leg.

The most important treatments for cellulitis of the leg are elevation and antibiotics. Unfortunately, both treatments are very difficult to carry out for the homeless patient living on the street. In severe cases, hospitalization may be necessary for leg elevation and intravenous antibiotics. Many of the homeless have no medical insurance, and hospitalization may not be an option unless the cellulitis is life or limb threatening. In severe cases, we try to get the patient into a shelter that has provisions for respite care. Respite beds in shelters are few, however, and we often settle for any indoor setting that allows the patient to elevate his or her leg.

Antimicrobial treatment for cellulitis must cover the most likely pathogenic organisms. An intravenous route is preferable, and the treatment of choice is a penicillinase-resistant synthetic penicillin (Sanford, 1989). A first-generation cephalosporin may be used in patients who are penicillin allergic.

Abscess

Fitzpatrick et al. (1987) define an abscess as "a localized accumulation of purulent material so deep in the dermis or subcutaneous tissue that the pus is usually not visible on the surface of the skin."

Infected intravenous drug injection sites are the most common cause of abscesses in the homeless. These abscesses are seen in the antecubital fossa but may present at any injection site. HIV infection must be actively considered in this setting.

S. aureus is usually the predominant infecting organism. Incision and drainage is the primary mode of treatment.

To perform this procedure, anesthetize the overlying skin with 1% lidocaine, and use a number 11 scalpel blade to make an incision over the abscess. Express the purulent material, and break down loculations with sterile cotton-tipped applicators dipped in hydrogen peroxide. Pack the cavity with (Nu-gauze) and schedule the patient back for follow-up in 1 to 2 days. Prescribe an oral antibiotic that has good antistaphyloccocal activity like dicloxacillin, erythomycin, or cephalexin.

Clean and repack the abscess cavity daily until drainage has mostly resolved. Then, instruct the patient in daily cleanings and dressing changes. Schedule for return visits or outreach visits as appropriate. The abscess should heal by granulation from the base up.

If the abscess is secondary to intravenous drug use provide AIDS counseling and HIV testing (with the patient's consent). If possible, offer the patient the option of entering a drug treatment program.

TRAUMA: LACERATIONS, BITES, AND BURNS

Physical trauma to the homeless may result in dermatologic injuries such as lacerations, bites, and burns. For a broader discussion of trauma in the homeless see Chapter 9.

Lacerations

Knifings, beatings, muggings, and fights are frequently causes of lacerations in homeless persons. Many homeless patients are intoxicated with alcohol or drugs at the time of the trauma; however, sober victims of violence on the street, within shelters, or in SRO hotels is not uncommon. With prompt medical care, these lacerations can be cleaned and sutured. With adequate follow-up, they will heal well.

Often, the homeless person does not come to the health provider until it is too late to safety suture the lacerations. When lacerations are not sutured, the time for healing is prolonged. Secondary infection is common in this setting, but can be minimized with meticulous wound care and prophylactic antibiotics.

Tetanus immunization status should be determined on all patients with traumatic injuries. When there is any doubt about immunization status tetanus, immunization should be administered. A few patients may also require tetanus immune globulin (Centers for Disease Control, 1985).

Bites

The "clenched fist" injury is the most common bite wound seen in the homeless (see Figure 10.3) This injury occurs when a person hits another person in the mouth with a clenched fist. This resultant wound is particularly dangerous because the oral bacteria flora with which it has been inoculated may cause a deep tissue infection (e.g., septic, arthritis, or osteomyelitis). Clenched-fist injuries in which the laceraton has penetration beyond the epidermis are best treated with hospitalization and intravenous antibiotics therapy. Inadequate treatment can lead to permanent disability.

When treating these injuries good local care is essential. Tetanus prophylaxis should be administered based on the patients immunization history. The preferred antibiotic therapy has become oral amoxacillin (Augmentin) and clavulanate potasssium, or intravenous ampicillin (Unasyn) and sulbactam. Finally, elevation of the injured extremity improves healing. For a good review of the management of bites, see Goldstein and Richwald (1987).

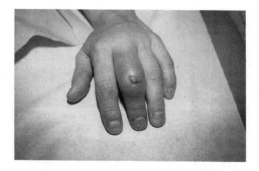

FIGURE 10.3 Cellulitis secondary to human bite wound—
"clenched-fist injury."

Burns

In our experience, the three most frequent causes of burns in the homeless are sunburns, burns from open fires used for cooking or heating, and intentional burns (usually inflicted on homeless persons sleeping in public places). Most homeless patients treated at the Venice Family Clinic have had first-degree or second-degree burns that do not usually require hospitalization.

The severest sunburns we have seen occurred when intoxicated homeless people fell asleep in the hot, Southern California summer sun. Infants and young children who have not been properly protected from the sun also are seen with severe sunburns.

Although less common, burns secondary to intentional violence do occur. One Venice Family Clinic patient, for example, had his sleeping bag set on fire while he was sleeping on the beach. Fortunately, he survived this attack with only second-degree burns that were treated at the clinic.

FUNGAL INFECTIONS

Fungal infections are prevalent among the homeless, the common organisms being *Candida albicans*, *Trichophyton* sp., and *Microsporum* sp. Tinea pedis is the most common type of fungal infection among the homeless because of the time they spend walking and because of poor foot hygiene (see Figure 10.4). A perfect environment for the growth of tinea pedis is established when feet, wet from the

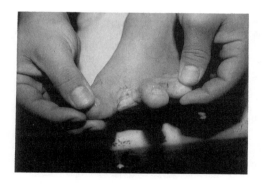

FIGURE 10.4 Tinea pedis—dermotophyte infection between the toes.

rain or perspiration, are not dried. The breaks in the skin caused by tinea pedis can lead to a bacterial superinfection and an ascending lymphangitis or cellulitis of the foot.

Other fungal infections in the homeless include *Candida vulvovaginitis, Candida balantis, Candida diaper dermatitis* in infants, onychomycosis, tinea cruris, tinea corporis, and tinea capitis. Many of these infections may be spread in overcrowded, poorly sanitized settings such as emergency shelters (see Figure 10.5).

Diagnosis of fungal infections is made by clinical appearance, potassium hydroxide smears from scrapings performed with the edge of a slide or a scalpel, and, when appropriate, fungal cultures. Treatment with topical antifungal agents may be adequate for tinea pedis and small areas of tinea corporis. Topical antifungal agents effective against dermatophyte infections (tinea) include miconazole (Micatin, Monistat), clotrimazole (Lotrimin), ciclopirox (Loprox), and tolnaftate (Tinactin). Tolnaftate is the only one of these agents that is not effective against Candida. Nystatin is highly efficacious against Candida but has no activity against dermatophytes. For large areas of tinea corporis and all cases of tinea capitis, oral griseofulvin must be used to eradicate the dermatophyte.

ECZEMA

The stress of homelessness and the irritants of the homeless person's environment may lead to severe exacerbations of chronic eczema. According to Fitzpatrick et al. (1983), "eczematous dermatitis is

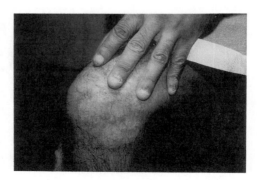

FIGURE 10.5 Tinea corporis (over the knee) and onychomycosis (fungal infection of the nails).

not a disease but a characteristic inflammatory response of the skin to multiple stimuli, both endogenous and exogenous."

Clinical types of eczematous dermatitis more commonly seen among the homeless include stasis dermatitis and lichen simplex chronicus.

The basic principles of therapy include the following:

- Avoid irritants to the skin. Remove potential contact irritants and use mild soaps or non-soap cleansers.
- Moisterize dry skin with ointments or emollients.
- Treat pruritis with antihistamines such as hydroxyzine or diphenhydramine.
- Apply topical corticosteroids to the affected area two times per day. The strength of the steroid should be increased as the severity of the dermatitis and the thickness of the skin involved increase.
- Use systemic antibiotics when the eczema shows signs of superinfection (wheeping, oozing, honey crusts, etc.).

An acute exacerbation of seborrhea may be a clue to the diagnosis of a new case of AIDS. Any acute seborrheic dermatitis in a patient at risk for AIDS should prompt further investigation (including an HIV antibody test). For further details on the diagnosis, classification, and treatment of specific types of dermatitis, see any general dermatological reference.

LICE AND SCABIES

Lack of hygiene, overcrowded sleeping accommodations, and sharing of clothes and bedclothes make the acquisition and spread of lice and scabies a frequent problem for homeless persons. Outbreaks of lice or scabies in shelters are common. It is not unusual for homeless persons to transmit lice or scabies from sharing blankets, clothing, or combs (especially among alcoholics). There are three types of lice: head lice–*Pediculus humanis capitis;* body lice–*P. humanis corporis;* and pubic lice (crab lice)—*Phthirus pubis.*

Lice

Head louse infestation is the most common infestation seen at the Venice Family Clinic among the homeless (see Figure 10.6). Itching is

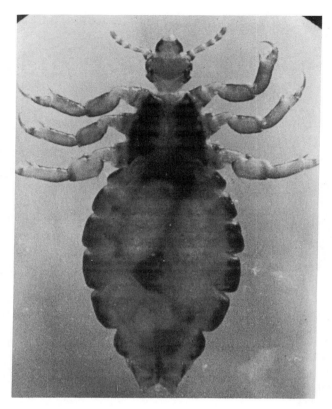

FIGURE 10.6 Head louse. (Courtesy of Reed and Carnrick.)

the most common complaint. The diagnosis of head lice is often made by finding the pearly white nits (eggs) glued to the shaft of the hair. These nits are most readily found among the hairs behind the ears and around the nape of the neck. In the typical infestation, the adult head louse is usually not seen. Occasionally we see a homeless person with an overwhelming infestation of head lice. In such cases, hundreds of adult head lice can be seen crawling all over the head, hair, and neck of the patient. This degree of infestation usually occurs only in the severely mentally ill, or in "down-and-out" alcoholics who have not shaved, bathed, or washed their hair in months. When the hair becomes matted with nits and covered with head lice, the patient must be given a short hair cut to eradicate the infestation. Medicated shampoo is still needed, but if the hair is not cut, shampoo alone will never cure such an infestation.

Pubic lice are also called "crabs" because their claws look like the claws of a crab (see Figure 10.7). They are usually spread by sexual activity, but can be spread by close nonsexual contact or through shared clothing or bedding. Crab lice often can be found attached to the pubic hair of the patient. Pubic lice eggs are brown and shiny and, therefore, more difficult to see than head lice nits. Because crab lice have a predilection for hairs of certain shaft diameters, they rarely live on the hairs of the head. Occasionally, they can be found on the hairs of the eyelashes, beard, axillae, lower abdomen, or thighs. When crab lice cannot be found, a presumptive diagnosis can be made if the patient has pubic itching and dark flecks of blood dotting his or her underwear. All patients with crab lice should be screened for other sexually transmitted diseases.

Body lice do not live on the body itself but in the seams of dirty

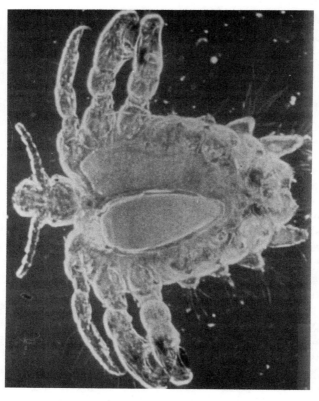

FIGURE 10.7 Pubic louse. (Courtesy of Reed and Carnrick.)

clothing. They leave the clothing approximately five times a day to feed on the blood of their human host. Body lice cannot be eradicated by cleaning the body alone. Body lice are killed by washing the infested clothing in hot water or going over the seams with a hot iron. Of course, discarding the old clothes for a new set of clean clothing may be a more practical alternative in some shelter settings. When body lice or their nits are found on the body, treatment is required.

Treatment for head, pubic, and body lice is essentially the same. The three major pediculocidal medications are 1% Gamma Benzene Hexachloride (GBH) Shampoo (Lindane, Kwell); Pyrethrin-containing shampoos (RID, A-200, Pyrinate); and 1% Permethrin Cream Rinse (Nix).[1] Because cure rates with 1% GBH and pyrethrins have been shown to be only about 60%, Kalter et al. (1987) suggest that a second treatment at 10 days should be routinely added for either pediculicide.

The manufacturers of Kwell or Lindane suggest the patient should lather the head or pubic hair for at least 4 minutes before washing off. Failures with Kwell and Lindane are probably secondary to incomplete ovicidal activity or reinfestation. These pediculocidal medications can be repeated in 24 hours but should not be used more than twice in 1 week. "While no evidence of toxic reactions has been described with use as directed by the manufacturer, some episodes of neurotic reactions, especially in infants, have been ascribed to Lindane misuse" (Kalter et al., 1987). Although Kwell is probably safe in children under age 2, the Pyrethrin or Permethrin preparations are recommended in this age group because of Kwell's potential neurologic toxicity.

The Pyrethrin preparations are applied to dry hair until it becomes entirely wet. After 10 minutes, the hair should be washed with water and any shampoo of choice. A second application should be made in 7 to 10 days to kill any newly hatched lice. The Pyrethrin preparations have the advantage of being over the counter and relatively inexpensive. They may be used for all types of lice and have no known significant toxicity if used as directed.

Nix is 1% Permethrin, which is a synthetic pyrethroid similar to natural pyrethrins. Nix is a cream rinse that is applied to the involved hair after it has been washed and towel dried. It is applied for 10 minutes and then washed out. Nix has the disadvantage of being more expensive than the other pediculicides because it is newer and has no generic competitors. Nix, like Kwell, also requires a prescription. In a study by Brandesburg et al., (1986). Nix demonstrated a higher 14-day cure rate for head lice than Lindane. Kalter et al. (1987), however, compared Nix with Lindane for the treatment of pubic lice and found no significant difference in the 10-day cure rates.

Regardless of the treatment chosen, head lice and eggs should be removed with a fine-toothed nit comb. Because none of the pediculicides are 100% ovicidal, it is helpful to remove any possible live nit from the hair. Because nits are cemented into the hairs, they may not come off easily. Dipping the comb in vinegar helps dissolve the cement and remove the nit.

All family members and close contacts should be examined and treated promptly to avoid reinfestation. Clothes and bedclothes should be washed in hot water. Contaminated articles such as hats and combs should be soaked in hot water for 10 minutes. Clinics should arrange for this service for their homeless patients. Shelter staff should also be alerted. When possible, they, along with outreach workers or public health personnel, should screen other residents of the shelter for infestations.

All lice infestations cause pruritus, which can lead to excoriations and secondary bacterial skin infections. When impetigo or other pyodermas are seen accompanying lice, they must be treated with appropriate antibiotics. Early treatment of lice can prevent these secondary bacterial infections.

Scabies

Scabies is a frequent infestation affecting the homeless. Persons with scabies come in complaining of an "itchy rash" that keeps them up scratching at night. They may even say the itching is so bad it is "driving them crazy" (see Figure 10.8).

Because the scabies mite is microscopic and not visible to the naked eye, making the diagnosis of scabies is more challenging than for lice. The first step in diagnosing scabies is to look for the typical skin lesions and the characteristic distribution of these lesions. Scabies can cause papules, vesicles, and burrows. Accompanying excoriations are secondary to the patient's scratching. These lesions are most commonly seen between the fingers, on the wrists, and in intertriginous folds of the axillae, groin, buttocks, and inframammary regions. Scabetic lesions may also be concentrated around the areolae of nipples in women and on the penis in men. Other areas of the trunk and extremities may be involved, but the face is almost always spared of lesions. Infants may have a more atypical distribu-

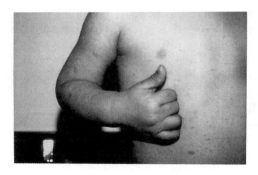

FIGURE 10.8 Scabies in a child. Child is scratching spontaneously.

tion with involvement of the face and head. Burrows are patho-gnomonic of scabies, especially when found between the fingers (see Figure 10.9).

It is helpful to find out if anyone else who has had close contact with the patient has a similar pruritic rash. If a whole family, a group of homeless companions, or a group sharing shelter space all have pruritic lesions with the morphology and distribution of scabies, then the diagnosis of scabies is certain. Scraping a burrow and finding the scabies mite or eggs under the microscope will confirm the diagnosis of scabies, but this procedure may be time-consuming and difficult to do. The yield on this procedure may be so low that scabies, for the most part, is a clinical, not a laboratory, diagnosis. With experience,

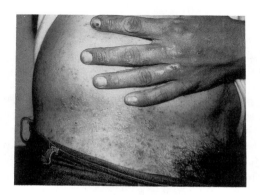

FIGURE 10.9 Scabies—pathognomonic burrow on middle finger.

making a diagnosis, based on history and physical examination becomes relatively quick and easy.

Until recently, scabies was treated with gamma benzene hexachloride lotion (Kwell, Lindane Lotion). This lotion is applied from the neck down for 8 hours. Kwell lotion is usually applied in the evening after a shower and washed off in the morning. It is important to instruct the patient to apply the lotion in all intertriginous areas, and between all the fingers and toes. Because access to a shower is an important issue for homeless persons, the timing of the application of Kwell may have to be modified. For example, in our clinic, we frequently allow patients to shower in our facilities during the afternoon homeless clinic and have them apply the Kwell Lotion immediately thereafter. Instead of keeping the Kwell on overnight, the patient returns to wash the lotion off during the evening clinic.

In addition to treating the patient's skin, it is essential to wash his or her clothes and linens in hot water. It is frequently more convenient to give the person "new" clean clothes.

For infants and children under 1 to 2 years of age with scabies, we recommended treatment with Crotamiton Cream (Eurax) to avoid the potential neurotoxicity that may occur with prolonged exposure to Kwell in this age group. The directions for Eurax are to apply the cream twice (24 hours apart) and to take a cleansing bath 48 hours after the first application. Because Eurax is probably less efficacious than Kwell, it may be necessary to repeat the treatment 1 week later if lesions and symptoms persist.

Recently, 5% permethrin (Elimite Cream) was approved by the Food and Drug Administration for treatment of scabies. *The Medical Letter* considers it the drug of choice for scabies (Medical Letter, 1990), since Permethrin appears to be safer than lindane. Elimite Cream has been approved for use in infants as young as 2 months. A number of studies have shown higher scabies cure rates with 5% Permethrin than lindane (Schultz et al., 1990; Taplin et al., 1986). The maufacturer of Elimite Cream recommends massaging the cream into the skin from the head to the feet, and leaving it on for 8 to 14 hours before washing it off. It looks as though 5% Permethrin will replace Kwell and Ewax for the treatment of scabies in the future.

The dead scabies mite under the skin is likely to cause continued pruritus for up to 1 week after any successful treatment. It is important to warn patients of this because an uninformed person may attempt to apply Kwell daily thinking that the initial treatment was ineffective. If applied daily, Kwell can cause an irritant contact dermatitis that complicates the picture. To give the patient symptomatic relief for the week following the scabicide application, prescribe antipruritic medications at the time of diagnosis and initial treatment, such as hydroxyzine (Atarax) or diphenhydramine (Benadryl) along with a topical agent such as 1% hydrocortisone.

Occasionally, a patient will have severe persistent itching beyond a week after a seemingly effective treatment. This could represent a treatment failure secondary to reinfestation from another person or the patient's environment. It could also represent incomplete application of the original scabicide. It is not unreasonable to repeat the Kwell, Elimite, or Eurax application at this time. However, The patient may have postscabetic syndrome, which is defined by unremitting pruritus, even after complete death of the scabies mite.

We treat postscabetic syndrome with systemic corticosteroids—40 mg of Kenalog intramuscularly for an adult; topical corticosteroids; systemic antipruritics; and topical Eurax twice a day for 5 days.

Schedule 1-week follow-up appointments for all patients treated for scabies. If the presumed scabies infestation is not improving, the clinician should consider the possibility that the original diagnosis may not have been accurate.

CONCLUSION

It is intellectually and emotionally challenging to provide health care to the homeless. By treating their dermatologic problems, we can provide relief from the annoying and painful symptoms that accompany skin disorders. Unsightly skin lesions on the face, hand, and body can also negatively impact on a homeless person's self-image. It is especially difficult to get a job with open sores on the face or hands. By treating and removing these oozing crusts or blemishes, we can temporarily help a homeless person's self-image and potentially aid his or her social function.

REFERENCES

Centers for Disease Control, (1985). Diphtheria, tetanus, and pertussis: Guidelines for vaccine prophylaxis and other preventive measures. *Morbity and Mortality Weekly Report, 34,*

Fitzpatrick, et al. (1983). *Color atlas and synopsis of clinical dermatology.* New York: McGraw-Hill.

Fitzpatrick, et al. (1987). *Dermatology in general medicine.* New York: McGraw-Hill.

Goldstein, & Richwald, (1987). Human and animal bites.

The Medical Letter on Drugs and Therapeutics. (1990, March). *Omeprazole.* New Rochelle, NY: The Medical Letter.

Kalter, et al. (1987). Treatment of pediculosis pubis. *Archives of Dermatology, 123,*

Sanford, (1989). *Guide to antimicrobial therapy.*

Schultz, M. W. et al. (1990, February). *Archives Dermatology, 126,* 167.

Taplin, D., et al. (1986). *Journal of the American Academy of Dermatology, 15,* 995.

Hypothermia and Exposure Among Homeless Persons

11

James R. Lockyer

CHAPTER HIGHLIGHTS

- Several factors increase the risk of hypothermia in the homeless: exposure to inclement weather, living conditions, infancy and old age, alcohol abuse, malnutrition, inadequate clothing and shelter, chronic illness, and mental illness.
- Mild and severe hypothermia can be confused with several other conditions common to the homeless population including alcohol or drug abuse and mental illness.
- Treatment for hypothermia is to raise the core body temperature slowly; the lower the core body temperature at the time of diagnosis, the more slowly the patient should be rewarmed.
- Most hypothermia patients should be referred to a hospital setting for a complete evaluation and continuous monitoring.
- Prevention is the best approach to hypothermia among the homeless and should be a priority of homeless health care programs all year long.
- One Los Angeles homeless outreach team has instituted a variety of hypothermia prevention measures: screening for high-risk patients; distribution of "cold packs"; development of good relations with other community service providers; provision of blankets and clothes; and communitywide shelter programs during cold weather.
- Cold packs, provided free to the homeless, contain articles essential to prevent hypothermia including a wool sock cap, multi-

vitamins with thiamine, a plastic ground tarp, an aluminum "emergency" blanket, and a printed education brochure on hypothermia prevention.

INTRODUCTION

Under normal conditions, the human body exhibits a remarkable homeostatic capacity to maintain a body temperature of 98.6° F ± 1°). Homeless persons are exposed to several factors that put them at high risk for hypothermia. This chapter describes these risk factors and the clinical manifestations and treatment of hypothermia. It concludes with several suggestions for preventing hypothermia in the homeless population.

RISK FACTORS AMONG THE HOMELESS

Several of the following factors increase the risk of hypothermia in the homeless:

- Exposure to inclement weather
- Living conditions that provide inadequate warmth and protection
- Infancy
- Old age
- Alcohol abuse (acute and chronic)
- Malnutrition
- Inadequate clothing
- Inadequate shelter
- Chronic illness
- Mental illness

The most obvious risk factor for hypothermia among homeless persons is their environment. For homeless persons, the risk of hypothermia changes with their living arrangement, which may change on a daily basis from a warm shelter to living on the streets, unprotected from the elements.

Although it is obvious that homeless persons are more at risk for hypothermia in cold weather, hypothermia can occur in any season including summer.

Most persons on the street are inadequately clothed, giving rise to a disproportionate degree of heat loss. In wet weather, body heat loss is magnified 20 to 30 times compared with dry conditions of the same temperature. Sleeping outdoors in direct contact with the ground also significantly increases heat loss. Furthermore, because homeless persons are frequently malnourished, their ability to generate heat and energy is impaired.

Up to 40% of homeless men abuse alcohol. Homeless alcoholics are at extremely high risk for hypothermia because they are commonly severely malnourished. Alcohol also causes vasodilatation and increased loss of body heat. Moreover, in an inebriated state, a person has an impaired sense of heat loss and cannot make decisions to seek a warm place or even put on more clothing. Lastly, chronic alcohol consumption depletes the body of thiamine, a vitamin that is essential for the normal functioning of the body's thermostat, the hypothalamus.

Approximately 40% of the homeless population suffers from mental disorders. Because the mentally ill are impaired in their ability to cope rationally with changes in their environment, they are also at high risk for developing hypothermia. Moreover, many homeless mentally ill on the street are taking neuroleptic medications, such as phenothiazines and tricyclic antidepressants, which impair the body's ability to respond to temperature fluctuations by conserving heat.

Medical conditions that predispose homeless individuals to hypothermia, even in the absence of cold weather, include congestive heart failure, chronic renal failure, cirrhosis, and endocrine disorders such as myxedema, hypopituitarism, and diabetes mellitus.

Studies demonstrate that, in their already compromised state of health, homeless persons are not only more susceptible to developing hypothermia, but are also more likely to suffer increased morbidity or die at each level of hypothermia. One study found that mortality rates for severe hypothermia increased from approximately 12% in otherwise healthy persons up to 48% in persons who had preexisting health problems.

CLINICAL MANIFESTATIONS OF HYPOTHERMIA

Persons suffering from mild hypothermia will exhibit dysarthria, shivering, ataxia, and moderate impairment of mental acuity. Despite these problems, they are usually oriented and responsive. It should be emphasized that the preceding findings may simulate drug or alcohol intoxication or severe mental illness. Therefore, clinicians must consider the possibility of coexistent or isolated hypothermia when evaluating homeless persons suspected to be intoxicated or severely mentally ill.

History

Typically, it is difficult to obtain a history directly from the patient owing to his or her impaired mental status. A history is, nevertheless, of critical importance. The history should include information regarding allergies, chronic illnesses, and medications the patient may be taking. In mild hypothermia, patients may explain that they are sleeping out of doors. Often, they will make a brief statement complaining of "feeling bad" or being unable to move, which they may repeat over and over again.

With further loss of body heat, a person will lose the ability to shiver. Movements will become progressively slower and stiffer, and the person will become more obtunded. Eventually, hypotension and bradycardia develop, and the person becomes comatose. Again, these signs are also consistent with alcohol or drug overdose, diabetic coma, a severe insulin reaction, head trauma, or the postictal state after a seizure. Thus, an appropriate medical history to rule out these conditions should be obtained from anyone available who knows the patient. Often, shelter providers, other service providers, or friends from the street can fill in important gaps in the medical history and provide information on the patient's risk factors for hypothermia.

Physical Examination

On physical examination, the most crucial pieces of information are the rectal or axillary temperature and vital signs (blood pressure and pulse). Hypothermia is defined as a body temperature of less than 95° F; it is clinically graded as mild (90° F to 95° F) or severe (below 90° F).The patient with severe hypothermia exhibits muscular rigidity, diminished or absent peripheral pulses, cool, pale skin, and decreased respirations. The patient may give the appearance of being dead. The patient may have myotic pupils and exhibit a diffuse edema. Deep tendon reflexes are also diminished or absent. A thorough physical examination should be performed to look for underlying causes of the person's hypothermia. Possibilities include antecedent trauma (especially to the head), evidence of drug abuse such as tracks, thyromegaly, skin and hair changes or other clinical findings consistent with thyroid dysfunction, evidence of congestive heart failure, or stigmata of chronic renal or liver failure.

Hypothermia can result in several medical complications whose presence or severity should be evaluated with laboratory examinations. In mild and severe hypothermia, metabolic acidosis develops as the result of excessive accumulation of lactic acid in the peripheral tissues. Blood gas and serum electrolytes will determine the degree of acidosis, and guide further therapy. Rhabdomyolysis may develop, and can be detected with an increase in the creatinine phosphokinase. Tissue destruction, compounded by hemoconcentration, may give rise to an elevation of the uric acid, blood urea nitrogen, and creatinine.

Victims of hypothermia often develop severe pancreatitis, which causes an elevation in the serum amylase. The patient may also exhibit stress-induced hyperglycemia or may present with profound hypoglycemia, presumably because of an impaired metabolism of circulating insulin. Hypoglycemia can cause significant morbidity or death, and should be evaluated immediately with a finger stick dextrostix.

TREATMENT OF HYPOTHERMIA

The immediate treatment objective is to raise the core body temperature slowly. Place the patient in a warm room, remove any wet clothing, and wrap him or her snugly (but not tightly) in warm blankets. If the person is comatose, an airway should be established. If the patient is conscious, they should be evaluated for a gag reflex, and given oxygen by mask or nasal cannula. Intravenous access should be established and baseline laboratory tests should be obtained including glucose, electrolytes, complete blood count, thyroid function, serum amylase, toxicity screen, and for other routine blood chemistries. All victims of hypothermia with impaired consciousness should empirically receive 100 mg thiamine intravenous push, followed by 50 ml of 50% dextrose intravenous push. They should also receive several ampules of naloxone, because a narcotic overdose may have been the precipitating event. A baseline 12-lead electrocardiogram should be obtained. This may exhibit the characteristic j-point waves known as "Osbourne waves" that are often observed in hypothermia. A chest radiograph should be obtained to assess the patient for possible congestive heart failure or aspiration pneumonia. The person should also be placed on a cardiac monitor for detection of cardiac dysrythmias.

It is not clear how aggressive further warming measures should be; efforts include administering warmed intravenous solutions, warmed aerosolized oxygen, and nasogastric and colonic irrigation with warmed fluids. The lower the core body temperature at the time of diagnosis, the more slowly the patient should be rewarmed. An abrupt rise in body temperature may induce a sudden increase in acidosis because of reperfusion of the acidotic peripheral tissues. This predisposes to potential malignant cardiac dysrhythmias.

Most hypothermia victims should be referred to a hospital setting for a complete evaluation and continuous monitoring. The only possible exception would be a patient with very mild hypothermia (94°F–95°F) who responds to therapeutic intervention with complete resolution of signs and symptoms. In these cases, the etiology of the hypothermia should be well characterized and self-limited (i.e., acute alcohol intoxication with exposure). In these circumstances, it may be appropriate to observe the patient for a period of 6 or 8 hours, and ensure that they are awake, oriented, well clothed and have access to food and shelter. The patient should be reevaluated on a daily basis for at least 2 to 3 days following the episode. Any question as to the cause of the hypothermia, or any complicating factors or problems requiring further evaluation warrants immediate ambulance referral to a hospital.

Measures to ensure follow-up of the patient after his or her release from the hospital might include direct instruction to the patient at the time of hospitalization as well as contacts with physicians, nurses, and social workers at the hospital. Encourage hospital providers to contact the clinic at the time of discharge to ensure follow-up care.

PREVENTIVE MEASURES IN PRIMARY CARE SETTING

Prevention is the best approach to hypothermia among the homeless. A formal program of hypothermia prevention should be developed by all clinics serving the homeless. The prevention of hypothermia is most important during cold weather, but it should be a priority all year.

Because the homeless at highest risk for hypothermia are often the least likely to seek evaluation on their own, an outreach program can prove helpful in identifying high-risk persons in the field. Outreach efforts include aggressively checking areas where people are likely to sleep out of doors, such as alleys and behind garbage dumpsters. A program of periodic visitation to hotels and shelters should be implemented to check on persons with known chronic disorders that predispose them to hypothermia. Outreach workers should also keep a careful watch for mentally ill and alcoholic patients. An outreach program also serves as a means of effective distribution of items such as a cold weather kit.

Following are listed several measures to prevent hypothermia instituted by the County of Los Angeles Skid Row Outreach Team, which primarily serves adult males in downtown Los Angeles.

- **Screening for High-Risk Patients**
  All clinic personnel are alerted to identify and provide additional assistance to those persons who are at highest risk for developing hypothermia including malnourished persons, alcoholics, the severely mentally ill, or those on antipsychotic medications.
- **Distribution of Cold Packs**
  The Los Angeles County Skid Row Outreach Program has developed an inexpensive packet that contains several articles essential to prevent hypothermia. Last winter, the Los Angeles City Police Department bought several thousand cold packs to distribute to the homeless throughout the city. The articles are small enough to fit into a plastic bag and include the following
  Wool sock cap—A disproportionately greater amount of heat loss from the head occurs because of the high volume of blood flow to the brain and scalp.
  Multivitamins with thiamine—These are especially important for the chronic alcoholic.
  Plastic ground tarp—This may be used as a ground cover or one may wrap their belongings and themselves in it to keep them dry.
  Aluminum "emergency" blanket—These compact blankets are sold at camping stores and are especially effective at retaining body heat.
  Printed brochure—These contain educational information on the risks and dangers of hypothermia, and provide useful tips on how to stay warm and how to use each item in the cold

pack. Brochures also include information on where to obtain free meals and shelter.

- **Development of Good Relationships with Other Community Service Providers**

  Communicating effectively with shelters and soup lines in your community will ensure that persons identified as high-risk for hypothermia receive assistance. For example, your clinic can prepare a letter to be given to persons with chronic ailments, such as diabetes. They can show the letter to shelter providers to ensure that they receive priority status in getting a bed for the night. Meal vouchers and bus tokens may also prove helpful.

- **Provision of Blankets and Clothes**

  Particularly when a person is intending to sleep out of doors, we provide them with blankets and warm clothing. Despite space limitations for storage, this is a very high priority at our clinic.

- **Communitywide Programs for Shelter Access**

  In periods of particularly cold weather, programs should be implemented that temporarily open additional congregate shelters for those who live on the street. In Los Angeles, a joint program of the city and county of Los Angeles transports homeless persons to National Guard Armories for 3-day stays during cold weather.

CONCLUSION

The homeless population living on the streets are at serious risk for hypothermia in almost all parts of the country, even in "sunny" Los Angeles. Through vigorous outreach efforts and coordinated temporary shelter programs during cold weather, homeless health care clinics and other service providers can significantly reduce the incidence of hypothermia in this population.

Tuberculosis in the Homeless

12

Claire B. Panosian

CHAPTER HIGHLIGHTS

- Tuberculosis is prevalent among the homeless population: Studies have found positive PPD skin tests in 18% to 51% and active tuberculosis disease in 1.6% to 6.8% of the homeless persons tested.
- The crowding and inadequate ventilation of many urban shelters, especially during winter months, enhances the potential for secondary spread of tuberculosis.
- New strategies for treating tuberculosis in the homeless population include multidrug short course regimens, an emphasis on education, screening, and a full range of case management activities.
- Homeless health care programs should establish educational tuberculosis programs for all employees and volunteers who work with the homeless.
- Intake histories of clients entering homeless shelters or clinics should include questions about prior tuberculosis exposure and tuberculin skin test results.
- All homeless individuals should receive an annual PPD to screen for recent tuberculosis exposure.
- Every asymptomatic homeless individual with a positive tuberculin skin test is a candidate for preventive isoniazid therapy, regardless of age.

- Whenever possible, homeless individuals with active tuberculosis should be given a 6-month multidrug treatment regimen. Twice-weekly, directly observed therapy instead of the standard regimen of oral medication is often necessary to ensure treatment compliance.
- Isolation, usually requiring hospitalization, is necessary with active pulmonary disease and positive sputum specimens.
- Homeless individuals with tuberculosis should not be allowed to return to a shelter or other communal residence until three consecutive daily sputum smears are negative.

INTRODUCTION

Before the advent of specific antituberculous pharmacotherapy in the 1940s, tuberculosis affected more than 100,000 Americans per year and claimed 40,000 lives annually. From 1953 to 1984, the prevalence of tuberculosis declined dramatically, with an average annual decrease of 5% in the number of reported tuberculosis cases. Along with the decline in active tuberculosis, the national pool of latent infected individuals also decreased. In contrast to a 50% rate of positive PPD skin tests in urban high school graduates at the turn of the century, it is now estimated that only 7% of the U.S. population currently harbor tubercle bacillus.

In the 1980s, however, another shift occurred. In 1985, for the first time in 30 years, the national incidence of tuberculosis stopped declining and plateaued at 21,801 cases, a rate of 9.1 per 100,000 population. In 1986, tuberculosis cases in the United States actually increased by 2.6% (Centers for Disease Control, 1989a). The most significant factor in this recent recrudescence is HIV-induced immunosuppression leading to reactivation of latent mycobacterial infection in previously asymptomatic hosts.

During the past several decades, the demographic profile of newly diagnosed tuberculosis cases has changed considerably. First, the minority population has experienced a less marked decline than the white population; at present, nearly two thirds of tuberculosis cases occur in minority groups (blacks, Hispanics, Asians, and Native Americans) as do 80% of all childhood cases (Centers for Disease Control, 1989). The higher risk for minorities is probably related in part to socioeconomic conditions such as inadequate nutrition, poor housing, and increased exposure to other infected hosts. Second, a steadily increasing proportion of cases occur in the elderly, independent of sex, or racial or ethnic background. Third, increasing numbers of cases are occurring in immunocompromised persons (i.e., HIV infection). Finally, immigrants, refugees, and migrant workers, whose country of origin has a high prevalence of tuberculosis, constitute a risk group for active infection with a greater than average likelihood of drug-resistant *Mycobacterium tuberculosis*.

Based on the shifting demographics of tuberculosis in the United States, it is easy to predict that this disease would disproportionately affect the homeless. Several overlapping risk factors for tuberculosis such as minority status, poor nutrition, alcohol and substance abuse, coexistent medical disease, HIV infection, and emotional stress are prevalent among the homeless population. Positive PPD skin tests have been found in 18% to 51% of homeless and indigent persons, and recent screening studies at clinics and shelters for the homeless have shown active tuberculous disease in 1.6% to 6.8% (Scheffelbein & Snyder, 1988; Slutkin, 1986). Although these data cannot be extrapolated to all subgroups of homeless (such as families with children and runaway children), they do indicate a prevalence of tuberculosis in some homeless patients that is 150 to 300 times higher than the national rate.

Housing conditions compound the risk of tuberculosis in homeless persons. The crowding and inadequate ventilation of many urban shelters, especially during winter months, enhances the potential for secondary spread of tuberculosis. Since 1984, at least six outbreaks of tuberculosis in shelters for the homeless have been reported to the Centers for Disease Control including one epidemic in Boston where a highly resistant strain was transmitted from a single index case to 49 other adults (Nardell et al., 1986).

Although the obstacles to tuberculosis control in the homeless patient are multiple, a recent heightened awareness of the problem and the unique features of tuberculosis management in the homeless patient are leading to new strategies. These strategies include education, screening, and a full range of case management activities.

The remainder of this chapter is devoted to an approach to tuberculosis in the homeless that encompasses the management of the individual patient as well as a description of systems and personnel that can collaborate toward the larger goal of eliminating tuberculosis from our society at large (Centers for Disease Control, 1989a; Scheffelbein & Snyder, 1988).

EDUCATION

All employees and volunteers involved in homeless health care need to be informed of basic facts about tuberculosis including its signs and symptoms, means of diagnosis, and treatment and prevention. This education should extend to shelter staff as well as medical service personnel. In addition, every homeless health care facility should have established lines of communication with the local health department; mechanisms for on-site PPD skin testing and sputum collection; rapid transport of specimens to an appropriate reference laboratory for mycobacterial stain, culture, and drug sensitivity testing; and convenient access to chest radiographs with on-site interpretation. Mycobacterial laboratories serving public hospitals and clinics should report positive sputum smear or culture results promptly (preferably by telephone if there is more than a 1- to 2-day delay in routine notification procedures).

Health facilities serving the homeless should routinely monitor their tuberculosis program and cases for appropriate diagnosis, treatment, public health department communication, and close follow-up. All positive PPD reactions must be evaluated. The local health department is responsible for treatment of all active cases and screening of known contacts. Unfortunately, a poorly implemented program will actually exacerbate our tuberculosis problem, because incomplete therapy encourages the development of drug-resistant *M. tuberculosis*, a lesson all too painfully learned in many developing countries of the world.

GENERAL TREATMENT GUIDELINES

Tuberculosis is a chronic bacterial infection that is spread from person to person by aerosolized respiratory droplets containing causative microorganism *M. tuberculosis*. Once inhaled, tubercle bacilli may lodge and replicate exclusively in the lungs, or disseminate throughout the body. Six to 14 weeks following primary infection, the typical human host develops tissue hypersensitivity to tuberculin proteins. This process is reflected in a positive delayed-type reaction to the tuberculin PPD skin test, a response that often persists for life. At the same time that the skin test converts to positive, newly activated immune cells in the human body contain the proliferation of mycobacteria.

Many otherwise healthy individuals with primary tuberculosis never manifest acute symptomatic disease, although their infection will continue for life. Other patients with long-standing latent infection experience endogenous reactivation and clinical illness after general host resistance declines because of age or other factors. The traditional risk factors for reactivation of tuberculosis are old age, malnutrition (often seen in chronic alcoholics), immunosuppression, diabetes, uremia, gastrectomy, and silicosis. In addition, there is now a significant association between tuberculosis and HIV infection, with reactivation tuberculosis often preceding other opportunistic diseases included in the diagnostic criteria for AIDS (Centers for Disease Control, 1986b, 1989a).

The diagnosis of tuberculosis is suspected when a patient with a positive skin test or suggestive epidemiological risk factors presents with a wasting febrile illness. Respiratory symptoms and chest radiographic abnormalities are the most frequent accompaniment to active infection, although extrapulmonary tuberculosis involving lymph nodes, pleura, genitourinary organs, bones, joints, and other organs occurs in 15% of all cases. Whatever the suspected site of infection, obtaining tissue or body fluid specimens (such as sputum, urine or pleural fluid) before the initiation of antituberculous therapy is essential. Children can rarely produce sputum, so a morning gastric aspirate culture for mycobacteria, although only 30% to 40% sensitive, is the best culture method. Because bacteriological diagnosis is very difficult in children, the diagnosis may rest almost exclusively on exposure history (Starke, 1988). However, whenever possible, specimens for culture and drug susceptibility testing should be obtained because of the growing number of single and multidrug-resistant strains of *M. tuberculosis*.

The pharmacotherapy of tuberculosis is a subject that can only be briefly summarized here; additional information is provided in standard treatment guidelines published by the American Thoracic Society (American Thoracic Society, 1986; Starke, 1988). For limited infection, which is evidenced only by PPD skin test conversion, a 6- to 12-month course of isoniazid alone affords up to 90% protection against future disease activity (Coleman & Slutkin, 1984). Clinicians should always balance the decision for preventive therapy with the potential risks of treatment, which include a rising incidence of isoniazid-associated hepatoxicity with age (2.3% incidence in patients 50 to 64 years old) and a variety of possible drug interactions with agents such as alcohol, phenytoin (Dilantin), and disulfiram

(Antabuse). Isoniazid-associated hepatoxicity is rare in children younger than 15 years of age, and unless there is a history of liver disease, screening liver function tests are not necessary. No patient should be placed on isoniazid prophylaxis without a screening chest radiograph and other laboratory investigations (urinalysis, lumbar puncture, node excision) needed to exclude the presence of more extensive tuberculous disease.

When clinically active pulmonary or extrapulmonary tuberculosis has been documented, several drugs in addition to isoniazid are commonly employed in combination regimens of 6 to 24 months' duration (American Thoracic Society, 1986). Because of the unusually slow multiplication of *M. tuberculosis*, it is always necessary to use at least two effective agents simultaneously to prevent the emergence of drug-resistant mycobacteria during therapy of active disease. The five drugs currently considered first-line antituberculous agents in the United States are listed in Table 12.1. Other drugs such as capreomycin, kanamycin, ethionamide, para-aminosalicylic acid, and cycloserine are used only in highly resistant cases under the supervision of a tuberculosis specialist.

Table 12.1 First-Line Antituberculous Drugs

Drug	Adult daily dosage	Pediatric dosage	Action	Toxicity
Isoniazid	300 mg[a]	10 mg/kg	Bactericidal	Liver, central nervous system, neuropathy, skin
Rifampin	600 mg[a]	15 mg/kg	Bactericidal	Liver, marrow, skin, kidney
Pyrazinamide	25 mg/kg	25–30 mg/kg	Bacteriostatic	Liver, gastrointestinal, uric acid
Ethambutol	15 mg/kg	[b]	Bacteriostatic	Eye, skin, uric acid
Streptomycin	15 mg/kg (intramuscular)	15–20 mg/kg (up to 1 g)	Bactericidal	Eighth nerve, skin

[a]Biweekly doses for isoniazid and rifampin are 900 mg and 600 mg for adults, and 20–30 mg/kg and 15 mg/kg, respectively, for children younger than 15 years old.
[b]Not recommended in children younger than 8 years old or children unable to perform color vision testing.

One well-validated regimen for treatment of uncomplicated tuberculosis is the combination of daily or biweekly isoniazid and rifampin for 9 months; in clinical trials, these two bacteriocidal drugs
given together produced relapse in only 1% to 2% of compliant users
with susceptible infections. There is now growing enthusiasm both
internationally and nationally, however, for an even shorter 6-month
regimen consisting of isoniazid, rifampin, pyrazinamide, and ethambutol or streptomycin given daily under close supervision for 2
months, followed by an additional 4 months of isoniazid and rifampin. This intensive multidrug program is advantageous because it
provides rapid sterilization of contagious infections while minimizing the potential for relapse even when drug-resistant mycobacteria
are present.

CASE MANAGEMENT

Screening

Because of the high rate of prior tuberculosis exposure among
homeless individuals, tuberculin skin testing is crucial to tuberculosis control in this group. The U.S. Public Health Service now recommends that all U.S residents have at least one PPD skin test result in
their medical records (Centers for Disease Control, 1989a). Homeless
persons have worse access to health services and are less likey to have
had a screening PPD. One recent Seattle study, for example, found
that only 27% of children of sheltered homeless families had ever
received a tuberculosis skin test compared with 48% of the U.S.
general pediatric population (Miller & Lin, 1988).

Ideally, all intake histories of clients entering homeless shelters or
clinics should include questions about prior tuberculosis exposure
and tuberculin skin test results. A screening PPD should be performed during an initial visit. For the reasons listed earlier, homeless
individuals are at high risk for tuberculosis exposure during their
homelessness. Therefore, they should receive an annual PPD to screen
for recent exposure.

Because intradermal induration must be assessed 48 to 72 hours
after placement of the skin test, the initial communication with the
homeless client must instill rapport and assure a means of follow-up
contact. In a debilitated or malnourished individual, it may also be
necessary to place one or more control skin test antigens (such as
mumps or Candida), because these patients can have general skin test

anergy (nonreactivity), which would invalidate the significance of a negative tuberculin reaction.

We recommend that shelter staff, or any other personnel exposed to a population with greater than 5% prevalence of tuberculosis infection, should also undergo annual tuberculin skin testing.

Preventive Therapy

Every asymptomatic individual with a positive tuberculin skin test is a candidate for preventive isoniazid therapy, regardless of age. In particular, treatment should be strongly considered in PPD reactors with the following conditions: recent conversion from a negative to positive skin test; chest radiograph consistent with old pulmonary tuberculosis (with negative sputum smears and cultures); and any medical condition known to increase the risk of active tuberculosis, such as alcohol or drug abuse, malnutrition, immunosuppressive therapy, HIV infection, gastrectomy, or silicosis. The final decision for treatment should ultimately rest with a qualified medical provider who can fully analyze the potential risks and benefits of treatment.

When patients are begun on isoniazid, the need to complete a full course of therapy (6 to 12 months) should be frankly discussed with the patient. With homeless individuals, it is often preferable to ensure compliance by means of twice-weekly, directly observed therapy instead of the standard regimen of daily isoniazid. If this is not possible, patients should be monitored at regular monthly intervals for signs and symptoms of toxicity, and compliance assessed by spot testing of urine for isoniazid metabolites.

On rare occasions, it is necessary to treat a person who has been recently exposed to a patient with active tuberculosis infection known to be isoniazid resistant. In this situation, three alternatives exist: prescribe isoniazid in the hope that it will still control infection in the second host; prescribe another drug regimen such as rifampin with or without ethambutol; or withhold preventive therapy and observe. For a high-risk contact, many infectious disease clinicians would adopt the second course of action and use alternative therapy to isoniazid in standard doses for 12 months.

Active Tuberculosis

When tuberculosis is strongly suspected on clinical grounds, the homeless patient will often benefit from hospitalization with respiratory isolation to expedite the diagnostic evaluation, prevent further transmission, and begin therapy promptly under medical supervision. If outpatient rather than inpatient evaluation of suspected tuberculosis is elected, careful record keeping, follow-through, and close contact with the client is necessary. Delays or failure to initiate treatment may result in a continuing risk of tuberculosis exposure to other clients and shelter staff as well as a direct threat to the health of the patient.

Within 4 days of the diagnosis of active tuberculosis, each patient should have an individualized treatment and monitoring plan and a specific health department staff member assigned to provide education and ongoing contact. As in all homeless health care, the clinical staff and case manager should maintain a nonjudgmental and supportive attitude. Incentives to enlist the cooperation and trust of the patient, ranging from clinic transportation to the provision of coffee, food, or personal items, are recommended. Probably the most important incentives are a warm, trusting relationship with the client and the removal of barriers to care. Visits to the homeless person's shelter or living locale assist in this process. All tuberculosis care and prescribed drugs should be provided free of charge.

The specific treatment of a homeless patient with active tuberculosis cannot be fully summarized here, but, whenever possible, a 6-month multidrug regimen should be employed. Ideally, this approach would involve a 2-month period of supervised daily therapy with isoniazid, rifampin, pyrazinamide, and possibly ethambutol, followed by an additional 4-month course of daily or twice-weekly isoniazid and rifampin. If daily observation during the first 2 months of treatment is not feasible, an alternative strategy is directly supervised therapy 3 days per week using the same initial drugs but higher dosages of isoniazid (15 mg/kg), pyrazinamide (up to 2.5 g), and ethambutol (30 mg/kg). In this protocol, the dose of rifampin is not altered despite the longer interval of administration.

Clinical and laboratory monitoring is another important aspect of active tuberculosis management. Baseline liver function tests should always be obtained before the institution of antimycobacterial drugs in adults and repeated at regular intervals depending on the patient's clinical status and relative risk of hepatotoxicity. For patients with pulmonary tuberculosis, sputum smears and cultures are repeated every 2 to 4 weeks until they become negative. No infected patient should return to a communal residence until three consecutive daily sputum smears are documented to be negative. This usually requires the health care team to arrange respite care or hospitalization for the patient until sputum smears are negative.

Finally, in the rare instance when an infectious patient refuses to comply with therapy and isolation precautions, quarantine measures including temporary institutionalization or court-ordered compliance with directly observed therapy are fully justified for the patient's health and the protection of others.

Contacts and Prevention

According to the U.S. Public Health Service standards, close contacts of persons with active tuberculosis infections should be examined within 7 days of the diagnosis of the index case. Contacts include those persons who are living in close proximity to the index case. If there is no evidence of clinical disease in the contact, the decision for preventive therapy with isoniazid or another agent is usually dependent on the tuberculin skin test status of the contact and other medical risk factors. Children who are household contacts of an infected patient, despite the presence of a negative skin test, are often placed on isoniazid preventive treatment, and reassessed at 3 months. If, at that time, the PPD is negative, isoniazid therapy can be stopped; if the child converts to a positive PPD test, he or she should receive a full 9- to 12-month course as well as a screening chest radiograph.

In addition to the principles of case finding and case management outlined earlier, some experts suggest the use of ultraviolet lights to reduce the transmission of tuberculosis in selected shelter situations, particularly those that are crowded and poorly ventilated. Currently, no epidemiological studies have evaluated the efficacy of this intervention.

CONCLUSION

In summary, the most successful strategy for the containment and ultimate elimination of tuberculosis in the United States is early case finding and completion of effective treatment regimens by infected individuals. This is a special challenge when dealing with persons who are without a fixed residence and struggling with the exigencies of daily survival.

REFERENCES

American Thoracic Society. (1986). Treatment of tuberculosis and tuberculosis infection in adults and children. *American Review of Respiratory Disease, 134*, 355–363.

Centers for Disease Control. (1989a). A strategic plan for the elimination of tuberculosis in the United States. *Morbidity and Mortality Weekly Report, 38* (Suppl. S-3),

Centers for Disease Control. (1989b). Tuberculosis and human immunodeficiency virus infection: Recommendations of the Advisory Committee for the Elimination of Tuberculosis (ACET). *Morbidity and Mortality Weekly Report, 38*, 236–250.

Coleman, D. L., & Slutkin, G. (1984). Chemoprophylaxis against tuberculosis. *Western Journal of Medicine, 140*, 106–110.

Miller, D. S., & Lin, E. H. B. (1988). Children in sheltered homeless families: Reported health status and use of health services. *Pediatrics, 81*, 668–673.

Nardell, E., McInnis, B., Thomas, B., et al. (1986). Exogenous reinfection with tuberculosis in a shelter for the homeless. *New England Journal of Medicine, 315*, 1570–1575.

Scheffelbein, C. W., & Snyder, D. E. (1988). Tuberculosis control among homeless populations. *Archives of Internal Medicine, 148*, 1843–1846.

Slutkin, G. (1986). Management of tuberculosis in urban homeless indigents. *Public Health Report, 101*, 481–485.

Starke, J. (1988). Modern approach to the diagnosis and treatment of tuberculosis in children. *Pediatric Clinics of North America, 35*, 441–464.

Pediatric and Maternal Health Issues

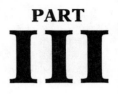

Obstetrical Care and Family Planning for Homeless Women

13

Elizabeth McNally, Julie Wood

CHAPTER HIGHLIGHTS

- All pregnancies in homeless women are considered high risk because pregnant women lack stability and a social support system, obtain late or no prenatal care, have poor nutritional status, and often suffer from mental illness and drug or alcohol abuse.
- Assessment of homeless pregnant patients should include histories of the present pregnancy as well as past gynecological, medical, and family problems.
- Accurate pregnancy dating may frequently require a prenatal ultrasound.
- Pregnant homeless women should be evaluated for alcohol and drug use, AIDS, and other STDs.
- Several medical and obstetrical problems found in homeless pregnant women require referral to high-risk obstetrical clinics. Much of the care for this population, however, can be managed by homeless health care clinics alone or in partnership with a tertiary care center.
- Homeless pregnant women should be seen often, at least biweekly during the first two trimesters of pregnancy and weekly thereafter.
- Providers should actively screen for early signs of common com-

plications of pregnancy such as preeclampsia, diabetes, high blood
pressure, and premature labor.
- Education, including family planning options, are an integral
  part of each pregnancy visit.
- Homeless pregnant women are best served by a multidisciplinary team that includes clinic-based and outreach personnel, and provides case management services.
- Public health nurses can effectively provide outreach services
  and postpartum follow-up visits in homeless shelters.

INTRODUCTION

Pregnant homeless women pose a unique challenge to the health
care delivery system because of the high-risk nature of their pregnancies and the environment in which they live. Health care providers
must work as a team and make special efforts to address the social,
economic, and medical problems of pregnant women if these women
are to have a chance of giving birth to a healthy baby. This chapter
first provides information on the risk factors associated with pregnancy among homeless women and the appropriate history, physical,
and laboratory assessment that should be undertaken. It then dis-
cusses follow-up and outreach efforts needed to help homeless
women maintain contact with the health care system during pregnancy. The chapter concludes with a case study demonstrating how
special efforts on behalf of these women pay off in the birth of a
healthy child.

RISK FACTORS AMONG
PREGNANT HOMELESS WOMEN

All pregnant, homeless women are considered high risk because
they lack a stable home and social support system, obtain late or no
prenatal care, have poor nutritional status, and often suffer from
mental illness and drug or alcohol abuse.

Lack of a stable home makes it difficult for homeless women to
obtain prenatal care. Forced to move from shelter to shelter, sometimes to escape from abusive relationships, pregnant women have
little time to worry about making or keeping prenatal care appointments. Once life is established in a new shelter, a pregnant woman

may be quite far away from her primary medical care site. Problems of transportation and day care for other children further hamper efforts to obtain prenatal care.

Homeless pregnant women are also at risk because of poor social supports. They are frequently alone and without any friends or family, except their own young children. They live in a stressful environment and must care for their children in the midst of crisis. It is rare for these women to have time alone. Shelters provide little emotional support during the difficult and uncomfortable times of pregnancy. Often, even when a husband or boyfriend is present, he provides little or no social or economical assistance, and may actually be depending on her welfare check for his own financial support. This is especially true when one or both parents are using drugs.

Late prenatal care is common among homeless women. It is not unusual for a pregnant homeless woman to walk into clinic 7 to 8 months pregnant, having received no prenatal care. Generally, these women are quite transient and have not stayed long enough in any one area to begin prenatal care. They come to the clinic because they are nearing their due date, or because they need a pregnancy verification to qualify for welfare benefits. Often, these women are unsure of the date of their last menstrual period, which makes it difficult to evaluate fetal growth and maturity.

Homeless women are at high risk for nutritional problems during pregnancy. A Nutrition Task Force of the American College of Obstetricians and Gynecologists has determined that the following circumstances and conditions, all of which are common among homeless women, are likely to compromise nutritional status:

- Economic deprivation
- Closely spaced pregnancies
- Smoking, drinking, or drug use
- Low weight at the beginning of pregnancy
- Anemia (hematocrit below 33%)
- Poor weight gain (less than 2 pounds for any month during the second or third trimesters)

Prenatal care experts recommend a caloric increase during pregnancy of 300 kcal/day. Because many shelters and soup kitchens serve only one or two meals daily, homeless women may have difficulty achieving this calorie intake. Moreover, shelter meals often consist of low-calorie or nutritionally imbalanced foods. Vitamin and iron supplements, and WIC coupons for supplemental food, which have been shown to be beneficial in improving the diet of poor women, are often inaccessible to the homeless because of their transiency and lack of prenatal care.

Mental illness in homeless pregnant women poses a great challenge to health providers. Mentally ill women may present to clinics in the third trimester without any previous prenatal care. Their chief complaint is often unrelated to pregnancy, and when confronted with their pregnancy, they often deny it. The clinician can become extraordinarily frustrated, trying to care for a woman who is 7 months pregnant, living on the street, and refusing to believe that she is pregnant.

In extreme situations, when a mentally ill pregnant woman is considered a threat to herself or a threat to the viability of her fetus, involuntary placement in a mental health facility may be required. The following case illustrates this situation.

> A 45-year-old black woman arrived at a clinic complaining of a cold and sore throat. She was about 34 weeks pregnant. When questioned about her pregnancy, she denied it. Instead, she smiled, sympathetic to the "practitioner's fantasy," and declared, "That is just my nerves." Her "voice" ordered her out of each of the shelters and SROs in which she had been placed. When she lost approximately 12 pounds in a 3-week period, and was heard talking about "something living inside me that needs to be cut out," we planned to commit her involuntarily. Fortunately, she agreed to hospitalization on her own. She remained hospitalized for the duration of her pregnancy (6 weeks) on an open psychiatric ward. Following birth, the baby was placed in foster care, but permanent placement for the woman is still being sought.

Finally, drug abuse, which is common among homeless women, further increases the risk for poor pregnancy outcome. The most commonly used drugs among homeless women are alcohol, crack cocaine, heroin, PCP, and amphetamines. Problems associated with drug or alcohol use in pregnancy are noncompliance with prenatal care, poor nutrition, fetal alcohol syndrome, STDs, intrauterine growth retardation, preterm labor, stillbirth, low birthweight, and infant withdrawal. Newborns may be irritable, feed poorly, and cry continuously. Longitudinal studies have also found that the children of mothers who abused drugs or alcohol during pregnancy suffer from developmental delay, concentration deficits, and aggression.

ASSESSMENT OF THE
HOMELESS PREGNANT PATIENT

History

The initial clinic interview of a new homeless prenatal patient should include questions about her living circumstances, such as the place she slept last night, where she "hangs out," and current contacts with social service agencies. The interview should be conducted in privacy, and questions should be kept simple. Patience, and a willingness to wait for responses, will help in establishing a trusting relationship with a homeless client who might be suspicious or even fearful of professionals.

A complete risk assessment must include information regarding each past pregnancy: miscarriages, abortions, weeks of gestation, length of labor, spontaneous or induced labor, type of delivery, baby's viability and weight, and maternal and neonatal complications. Information should also be elicited regarding the present pregnancy and the gynecological history, family history, and medical history. It is very important to try and obtain the exact date of the patients last menstrual period. Combined with the fetal size measurements, one can accurately establish the length of gestation. Table 13.1 presents a list of topics or problems within each area that should be explored during the initial interview.

Drug Use Evaluation

Because of the multiple risks of drug abuse to the fetus, and the high prevalence of drug abuse among homeless women, each pregnant homeless woman must be thoroughly evaluated for drug use. Most patients deny or report only light use, even when they are heavy users. Because alcohol or drug use is often a predisposing factor for homelessness, however, the practitioner should always look for covert signs of abuse. Each client should be questioned directly and specifically about alcohol or drug use. All pregnant women should receive a urine screen for common illicit drugs, even if they deny drug use.

The interview and screening tests should look for the use of multiple drug types because most drugs are used in combination with others, such as cocaine and alcohol. Ask about the mode of use—do they smoke it, shoot it, or snort it? If a woman admits to past drug

Table 13.1 Obstetrical History

Present pregnancy history	Gynecological history	Family history
Bleeding	Menarche	Hypertension
Nausea, emesis	Menstrual amount,	Renal disease
Edema	duration, pain	Diabetes
Constipation	Intermenstrual bleed-	Malignancy
Pain	ing	Tuberculosis
Urinary tract infec-	Leukorrhea	Psychiatric problems
tion	Contraception	Multiple pregnancy
Headache	Infertility	Bleeding
Emotional	Abnormal Pap smear	Genetic abnormalities
Smoking		Genital herpes
Alcohol		
Drugs		
Medical History:		
Rheumatic fever	Anemia	
Hypertension	Epilepsy	
Kidney disease	Syphilis	
Diabetes	Gonorrhea	
Heart disease	Migraine	
Tuberculosis	Psychiatric problems	
Injuries	Transfusions	
Allergies	Endocrine	
Current medications	Drug addiction	
Operations		

abuse, question her about how she quit. Rarely does anyone get off alcohol, crack cocaine, or heroin without going through a rehabilitation program. Suspect continued use if a patient says she "just stopped on my own."

Homeless women with a history of drug use during the present pregnancy (even if they stopped in the first trimester) should be referred to a high-risk obstetrics clinic for more intense fetal evaluation. The woman should receive education about the effects of drug use on the fetus, and also be encouraged to attend drug counseling or to enter a residential rehabilitation facility, if one is available. Pregnancy and the fear of losing the baby may be the needed impetus to stop using drugs.

Because of their drug use, however, some women will avoid prenatal care, fearing that a positive urine drug screen will cause them to lose custody of the newborn. Therefore, it is important to reassure the woman that the clinician's goal is to help the woman "get clean" and to produce a healthy infant. Legally, even if she has positive urine drug screens early in pregnancy, but is able to produce negative urine screens in the third trimester and at delivery, she will go home with the newborn; a positive drug screen at birth will mean certain loss of custody, at least temporarily.

A woman with a positive urine drug screen during the third trimester should be reported to Children's Protective Services as endangering her fetus. She should also be reported, with due date, to the local hospital's obstetric and social work departments. The social workers should then notify the labor and delivery staff, so that a drug screen and proper intervention will occur at birth.

If a newborn is taken away from the mother at birth, the public health nurse or social worker can act as liaison with children's services, helping to enroll the mother in a drug rehabilitation program and monitoring her progress in staying off drugs—requirements she must meet to get her child back. They can also assist with parenting classes and drug rehabilitation programs.

Any woman suspected of intravenous drug use, prostitution, or whose spouse is an IVDU, should have HIV antibody and serum hepatitis B antigen testing. An HIV test requires a special consent from the client and precounseling and postcounseling. All records and HIV test results must be kept confidential. If either test is positive, the patient should be referred to the high-risk obstetrics clinic. HIV and hepatitis B screening is now done routinely as part of the prenatal care for all homeless prenatal patients.

High Risk Referrals

Because many homeless women have high-risk pregnancies that require specialty care, neighborhood clinics serving the homeless need to establish a contractual relationship with a nearby hospital to assure that it will accept clinic referrals for pregnant women. Table 13.2 presents risk factors that determine referral to a hospital's high-risk obstetrics clinic.

Table 13.2 High-Risk Pregnancy Criteria: Indications for Specialty Obstetrical Referral

Medical	Obstetrical
Anemias (unresponsive to iron)	History of previous stillbirth or
Gestational diabetes	neonatal death
Pyelonephritis	History of previous infant under
Epilepsy	2,500 g
Hypertension	History of habitual abortion
Genital herpes	History of previous cesarean sec-
Drug abuse	tion
Person's refusing blood transfusions	Previous difficult delivery
Insulin-dependent diabetes	Intrauterine growth retardation
Cardiac disease	Genetic problems—strong family
Renal disease	history
Hyperthyroidism	Twins
Collagen vascular diseases	Oligohydramnios or polyhydram-
	nios
	Preterm labor
	Vaginal bleeding
	Postdate (42+ weeks)
	RH or other sensitization
	Abnormal Pap smear
	Patients needing amniocentesis

When a patient has a high-risk pregnancy, but is not experiencing any symptoms of acute problems, the neighborhood clinic practitioner can perform a comprehensive assessment including a history, physical examination, pelvic examination, and blood work before sending the patient to a hospital high-risk obstetrics clinic. Furthermore, the neighborhood clinic practitioner often may continue to follow many high-risk pregnancies jointly with the obstetrics specialists. Patients benefit from receiving their prenatal care locally because many lack funds for transportation and are frightened by large hospital facilities. Personal, competent care received at a local clinic can be a strong complement to specialty obstetrical care. When followed at the local clinic it is possible to track patients that missed their routine appointments. The clinic should screen all missed and canceled appointments for high-risk patients. The clinic should then make every effort to bring the client in, such as messages with the day shelter, postcards to last known address, or use of the outreach team. In our experience the team approach with close follow-up greatly increases patient compliance and improves pregnancy outcome.

Frequently, neighborhood clinics see obstetrical patients who require immediate referral. The following are conditions that should be sent immediately to a hospital labor and delivery, or emergency department:

- Suspected labor, term or preterm
- Premature rupture of membranes
- Significant vaginal bleeding
- Preeclampsia-diastolic blood pressure > 95 mm Hg or significant proteinuria ($\geq$ 2+) or untoward symptoms (severe headache, epigastric pain, etc.)
- Serious acute illnesses, especially those that are apt to require hospitalization such as pyelonephritis, pneumonia, appendicitis, and so on
- Breech or transverse lie at 37 or more weeks

Physical Examination

In homeless women, the antepartum physical examination is similar to a regular antepartum physical, except that clinicians should also specifically look for skin popping or track marks on arms, groin, legs, or breasts; bruises suggestive of battering; altered mental status; signs of drug influence; and signs of alcohol intoxication or alcoholism. The pelvic examination should routinely include culture for gonorrhea and chlamydia. A wet mount for Trichomonas, Candida, and clue cells (nonspecific vaginitis) is also necessary since these infections are commonly seen in homeless women. Many Pap smears performed on homeless women have a diagnosis of mild atypia. In most cases, when appropriate treatment is rendered, the repeat Pap will be negative. If the pap returns with mild atypia after treatment, the patient is referred to the gynecologist. Condyloma acuminatum is also a common finding on examination of the vulva, vagina, and cervix. Small isolated condylomata are treated with trichloroacetic acid, whereas large, rapidly growing condylomata are referred for cryocautery.

Laboratory Assessment

Laboratory assessment should include a clean-catch urine sample to check for glucose, protein, white cells, and bacteria. As noted earlier, a urine toxicology screen is recommended for all women suspected of drug use. Serum antibody screen, blood type and Rhesus factor, rapid plasma reagin test, rubella, and hemoglobin are routine. A routine ultrasound is done between 16 to 20 weeks to assess fetal age. A 1-hour glucose tolerance blood test is done at 26 weeks. Hemoglobins are repeated about every 2 months. Many homeless women experience one to two urinary tract infections or episodes of bacteriuria that increase the risk for acute pyelonephritis and possible intrauterine growth retardation or prematurity. At times prophylactic treatment may be required for the duration of the pregnancy. When several episodes are documented, the patient must be evaluated further in a high-risk obstetrics clinic.

The same behaviors that make homeless pregnancies high risk—intravenous drug use, multiple sexual partners, and prostitution—also make homeless women at high risk for AIDS and other STDs. All pregnant clients entering the clinic should receive hepatitis and AIDS prevention education.

FOLLOW-UP DURING PREGNANCY

We recommend more frequent clinic visits for homeless women in the first two trimesters than is generally recommended (biweekly instead of monthly) and weekly thereafter. With their multiple psychological and social needs, homeless women can benefit from the extra contact, education, and case management provided at each visit. All homeless women should be referred to a social worker or public health nurse for psychosocial evaluation and case management.

At 36 weeks the presenting part is checked, and at 37 weeks, if the baby is breech the mother is sent to the hospital for version. If a woman goes beyond her expected date of confinement or due date, she should begin nonstress testing, and be given a fetal movement index chart to keep and record movements. She should be seen at the clinic every 2 days. At 42 weeks, a contraction stress test should be done at the hospital and induction considered.

At 32 to 34 weeks, contraception should be discussed in depth.

Tubal ligation should also be discussed and offered. Women do not usually consent to this procedure until after the third or fourth child, however. If a woman does decide to have a tubal ligation, the clinic team should assist her with the paper work in time to have the procedure performed right after delivery. Most of the homeless pregnant women have tried many forms of birth control with little success. If not ready for the tubal ligation, many women will try birth control pills. Education of the common problems experienced with the pill can help the patient continue its use if one of these problems occurs. Intrauterine devices are sometimes requested by the patients. Because of cost considerations, however, they are not routinely used by most facilities and, therefore, seldom an option for a homeless patient. Diaphragms are encouraged postpartum; however, women using diaphragms are often uncomfortable with insertion or find that they are inaccessible when needed. Condoms and foam are strongly recommended for disease prevention. Having the male partner present and educating both partners on their use has been found to be helpful.

At 32 to 36 weeks the topic of breast-feeding should be addressed. Although, breast-feeding is regularly the recommended choice in most facilities, it may not be with homeless clients. If a client is using drugs or alcohol postpartum, then formula-feeding is encouraged. Because of the lack of privacy in large shelters, homeless women may feel more comfortable with formula feeding. Often forced to leave the shelters during the day, these women cannot find convenient places to breast-feed. Breast-feeding can be successful for many with appropriate education and assistance, however. Breast-feeding is important not just for the natural immunity given but for the low cost. Formula is scarce in the shelters, and it is difficult to give the baby any specific brand or type he or she may be accustomed to.

Some patients are unable to keep appointments. If we suspect the patient may not return for the scheduled appointment, we may give only 10 prenatal vitamins at a time and tell the client that she must return every 10 days for a refill. Prenatal vitamins are a very desired item. If we are treating bronchitis or a urinary tract infection, we may give only 2 days of medication at a time, requiring the client to return every 2 days for refill. In this way, we can be nearly certain to see the client again soon.

A combination appointment and walk-in system works well in a homeless clinic. Leaving a few slots everyday for walk-ins and emergencies has proven advantageous for everyone. Thus, if a prenatal patient thinks she may be in labor, is in pain, or experiencing bleeding, she can walk in and be seen immediately.

Prenatal education classes are an important part of pregnancy care for homeless woman. The Samaritan shelter in Denver has a group of volunteer nurses who conducts a series of prenatal classes for homeless women. Prenatal education includes diet; exercise; signs of problems; signs of labor; dangers of smoking, drinking, and drug use during pregnancy; infant care; AIDS; and birth control. A shelter provides transportation to the classes, significantly increasing attendance.

At the Stout Clinic, an innovative homeless health care program in Denver, the prenatal patients followed by the nurse practitioner are given her home telephone number at about 34 weeks. The patient is told to call with any questions regarding labor and delivery. When the patient does go into the hospital for delivery, the practitioner is called, and, if possible, attends the birth, providing support and acting as a coach. This is helpful both to the mother and the hospital staff. The Stout Street Clinic practitioners are known and welcomed at the hospital's labor and delivery ward. After delivery, the hospital social worker will make sure the mother and child are being discharged to a shelter or safehouse, not to the street. A postpartum visit can be arranged. If temporary shelter referrals are refused by the mother, child protective services must be contacted to report the mother for child neglect.

Outreach

Several homeless health care projects use outreach teams to bring pregnant women into care and follow up on those who do not keep their appointments. For example, each day, Stout Clinic's outreach staff, consisting of two social service workers, a mental health worker, and a substance abuse counselor, goes out and looks for people that need services. The team also tracks down patients that fail to appear for follow-up visits by checking all the spots the patient has stayed in the past month, talking to people on the street, and contacting shelters and day shelters. Often, pregnant homeless women are contacted through use of an outreach team. The team not only locates clients for follow-up but will also, when necessary, help them get to their appointment. If, for instance, a client is developmentally disabled or is too frightened to travel by bus for a hospital visit, the outreach team will arrange a meeting place and take the client to her scheduled appointment. Unfortunately, no matter how compulsive one may be in outreach and follow-up, some clients are lost.

Another model of outreach care to homeless women uses a public health nurse as the outreach worker. Maternal and infant health is a high priority for the public health nurse. Because the public health nurse spends time in the community—in homes, shelters, and on the street—she or he can provide a comprehensive assessment of homeless clients. Further, because public health nurses are out in the homeless community, they, like other outreach workers, are more approachable than the practitioner in the clinic.

An initial outreach visit by the public health nurse should include the patient's history, physical assessment, one-to-one education, appropriate referrals, and emotional support. The brief history includes gynecological and medical history, with a focus on high-risk factors that might need immediate referral.

A public health nurse can perform a physical assessment in the field. The assessment includes appearance, signs of drug abuse (e.g., cachectic appearance, dry, limp hair, poor hygiene); mental illness (inappropriate affect, poor hygiene); blood pressure; signs of edema; and a urine sugar and protein test. The physical evaluation should also include any other signs of disease or infection that might need intervention. Vitamins and iron should be given as soon as possible because of the significant risk of poor nutrition in this group.

The prenatal education offered should cover the topics of nutrition, danger signs in pregnancy, signs of labor, STDs, AIDS, and family planning methods. Clients should be encouraged to ask questions and written materials are provided for later reading.

In a shelter setting, where there may be several pregnant women, the PHN can provide classes on different topics such as pregnancy, child birth, and infant care. These classes will reinforce the one-to-one education and also provide a social setting for these women.

The public health nurse can also help refer the client to the welfare office, housing, food and clothing agencies, child care, mental health facilities, drug counseling, and so forth. Clients should be helped to make appointments and provided with explicit directions, and, when necessary, bus tokens to facilitate follow-through. The public health nurse can then act as liaison between the client and agency after contact is established.

The public health nurse should also provide emotional support to, and advocate for, the homeless woman. Ongoing concern and care, competent medical advice, and reminders about the next appointment may keep someone coming back for prenatal care or may be what finally convinces a woman to begin prenatal care. The following two case studies provide examples of the importance of the public health nurse as a link between homeless pregnant women and the clinic-based care they need.

A young pregnant woman living in a large family shelter was angry and hostile at the public health nurse's first shelter visit. She refused to talk and would only accept the vitamins and iron supplements. The public health nurse gave her the space she needed but at each shelter visit reached out to her. Finally, after several contacts by the public health nurse, the woman began asking questions about her pregnancy. Finding out that the woman was quite intelligent, the public health nurse provided books and literature about pregnancy. At each visit, the public health nurse encouraged the woman to come for prenatal care. Finally, the woman agreed and continued with her prenatal care until delivery.

Another woman was living in the community in a very unstable, violent situation. The public health nurse met this woman during a home visit to another pregnant woman. At first, this woman refused prenatal care because she was using crack cocaine and did not want to have her future child taken from her. After establishing a relationship with the woman, however, the public health nurse convinced her of the special drug clinic's desire to help her "get clean" before delivery—not to simply label her and remove her infant.

In each of these case studies, the women received surveillance for danger signs of pregnancy, education, visits, and medical referrals before reaching the clinic. This early intervention combined with clinic care resulted in better pregnancy outcomes.

CONCLUSION

Care for homeless pregnant women is optimally delivered by a multidisciplinary team that includes clinic-based and outreach personnel. Despite the frequent high-risk nature of homeless women's pregnancies, much of their care can be managed by primary care providers in coordination with tertiary referral centers. Support for homeless pregnant women can clearly influence pregnancy outcomes. One family illustrates this point particularly well.

The wife had three previous miscarriages and had given up hope of ever having a child. She was 34 years old, a heavy smoker, living an unstable life, and moving frequently with her husband in search of work. She came to the clinic for a pregnancy test and was found to be about 8 weeks pregnant. She was very pleased but nervous about losing this child. The staff helped place the couple in a long-term shelter, and the husband began working day labor jobs. The wife came to the clinic for all her prenatal appointments. She had the nurse practitioner's telephone number to call in the event of any problems. The husband came to every appointment that he was able to attend. The couple became very hopeful as the pregnancy progressed normally. They had a beautiful 5-pound baby girl with no complications. They attribute this child's life to the quality of the prenatal care and support they received. They told clinic staff that, "If we had all the money in the world, we could not have bought better prenatal care." We attribute their baby's life to their concern and compliance with all their prenatal appointments, as well as their stability in the long-term shelter. Six months later, the husband was still working, and the family was living in its own apartment. They have developed a sense of self-respect and pride.

Evaluation and Management of Homeless Families and Children

14

David Wood

CHAPTER HIGHLIGHTS

- Families represent the fastest-growing segment of the homeless population.
- Homeless families are likely to be from a minority population and headed by a single parent.
- Homeless families frequently report serious family problems including spousal abuse, child abuse, and drug use.
- Homeless children have high levels of acute and chronic illness, are likely to have behavior problems, perform poorly on the Denver Developmental Screening Test (DDST), and have academic difficulty in school.
- Homeless families often cite benign acute problems as the reason for a clinic visit. Each encounter, however, should include a history of preventive health care, developmental problems, school problems, medical problems, and past child abuse.
- Furthermore, objective assessment of each child should be conducted through careful family observation, a thorough physical examination and screening, and appropriate tests.
- Homeless families and children need the services of a multidisciplinary team that provides—through medical and social assessments—outreach, intensive follow-up, and help with basic needs and medical referrals.

INTRODUCTION

The family, defined as one or more adults living with a dependent minor, represents the fastest-growing segment of the homeless population. In New York City, individuals in families constitute 35% to 50% of the homeless (New York Coalition for the Homeless, 1986); in Los Angeles, approximately 40% of the city's 40,000 to 60,000 homeless are family members (U.S. Conference of Mayors, 1984, 1986).

The national increase in family homelessness is primarily a result of two converging economic trends. First, the supply of affordable housing in major cities has significantly declined because of rising housing costs (rents), cutbacks in federal low-income housing programs, and the replacement of low-cost housing by inner-city development (Hartman, 1983).

Second, family poverty has increased. In the past 10 years, public AFDC grants have decreased by 10% in real dollars (U.S. Congress, 1986). Moreover, the number of families dependent on minimum-wage jobs has grown dramatically. These factors have caused the number of families in poverty to grow by more than 40% between 1981 and 1985 (U.S. Congress, 1986).

As a result of the trends in housing and family poverty, more poor families compete for fewer low-cost housing units. Families with problems—drug abuse, poor interpersonal communication, family violence, or mental illness—are the most vulnerable and least able to compete in the housing market. Therefore, they are more likely to lose permanent housing and become homeless. If the trends in housing costs and family poverty continue, however, more and more functional poor families will join the ranks of the homeless.

This chapter first presents the findings of a study of 200 homeless families and children and 200 housed, poor families conducted by the author in Los Angeles, (Wood et al., 1989a). It presents information on the families' socioeconomic characteristics and structure, and the children's health, development, and behavior problems. Next, the medical evaluation and diagnostic and therapeutic considerations for homeless families and children are discussed. The chapter concludes with a case study exemplifying an approach to the evaluation and management of the homeless child and family.

SOCIAL-DEMOGRAPHIC CHARACTERISTICS OF HOMELESS FAMILIES

Most of the homeless families in the Los Angeles study were from minority populations (57% were black, 7.7% Latino, and 5.6% other minority) and headed by a single parent (53%). Homeless mothers were, on the average, approximately 29 years of age. Compared with poor families who had homes, the mothers were less likely to have received a high school education; 43% of homeless mothers had not finished high school compared with 28% of poor mothers who had homes (see Table 14.1).

Homeless families are often dysfunctional and report a high level of family problems: 34% reported spousal abuse, 28% reported child abuse, and 43% reported drug use. One third of homeless mothers reported drug use, including crack and heroin, and 14% had been hospitalized for a mental health problem (see Table 14.2).

The cycle of family dysfunction and poverty is evident in homeless families. Homeless mothers frequently find themselves in a family environment similar to the one in which they grew up. Substance abuse and family violence were commonly present in the homeless mothers' own family of origin. Fifty percent reported coming from families in which their parents were addicted to drugs or alcohol;

Table 14.1 Characteristics of Homeless Women in Families

Characteristic	Homeless families (%) (N = 196)
Maternal ethnicity	
Black	56.9
Non-Latino white	29.7
Latino	7.7
Other	5.6
Maternal educational level	
K to 11th grade	43
High school diploma or some college	57
Family structure	
Female head, single parent	52.9
Two parents	47.1
Among two-parent families couple together more than 1 year	83

Table 14.2 Percentage of Mothers Reporting Violence, Drug or Alcohol Abuse, Criminal Involvement, and Mental Health Problems

Family or personal problem reported	Homeless families (%) (N = 192)
Violence	
Mate abuses mother	34
Mate involved in criminal activity	29
Social service file opened for child abuse or neglect	28
Drug and alcohol abuse	
Mate abuses alcohol or drugs	43
Mother abuses drugs	32
Mental illness	
Mate is mentally ill	15
Mother has history of hospitilization for mental health problem	14

31% had been physically or sexually abused as children, and more than one third had been placed with relatives or in a foster care home (see Table 14.3).

Given their family background, it is not surprising that homeless mothers have only a tenuous support system to depend on in time of crisis. On average, homeless mothers had only 1.8 adult friends or family members they could rely on; two thirds of homeless mothers named only one or no adult supports (see Table 14.4). Approximately

Table 14.3 Percentage of Homeless Mothers Reporting Problems in Their Own Families of Origin

Problem reported by mother	Homeless families (%) (N = 195)
Mother's family of origin headed by single female	40
Mother's parents divorced or death of parent(s)	43
Mother's parent(s) abused drugs or alcohol	49
As a child, mother lived with a relative or in foster care	35
Mother was physically or sexually abused by parent(s)	31

Table 14.4 Number and Type of Social Supports Reported by Homeless Mothers

Average or number of adult supports named by mother (range) (N = 189)	1.8
Percentage of mothers reporting (N = 196)	
One or no adult supports	66%
Two or three adult supports	26%
Four or more adult supports	8%

one third of the mothers depended on their minor children for support. Fewer than one third named their own parents as support, indicating the degree of estrangement homeless families commonly experience from parents and grandparents.

ASSESSMENT OF HOMELESS CHILDREN

Physical Health Assessment

Homeless children have high levels of morbidity and ill health (Table 14.5). Seventeen percent of homeless children were rated to be in fair or poor health by their mothers. Mothers reported that their children experienced an average of 5.4 symptoms, two sick days, and one bed day during the past month, and about 5% were ill enough to be confined to bed 4 or more days.

Table 14.5 Reported Health Status Measures for Homeless Children

Health status measure	Homeless families (N = 194)
Percentage in fair or poor health	17%
Number of illness symptoms reported during past month (mean)	5.4
Percentage with 4 or more sick days during past month	16%
Percentage with 4 or more bed days during past month	5%
Percentage of parents worried about child's health	43%

During the past month, homeless children had high rates of common symptoms such as fever, cough or colds, and vomiting or diarrhea (see Table 14.6). The reported frequency of diarrhea during the past month was more than five times higher, and cold symptoms more than 50% higher than in the general child population. The month-period prevalence for asthma symptoms among homeless children was more than 10%, two to three times higher than in the other disadvantaged groups (Mak et al., 1982; Siegel, 1986).

Behavior Problems, Development, and School Performance of Homeless Children

Homeless parents commonly reported that their children had behavior problems such as frequently stubborn, sullen or irritable, hitting other children or adults, and frequent temper tantrums.

Homeless children performed poorly on the DDST (Jaffe, Harel, Goldberg, et al., 1980); 9% of the children failed two or more sections on the DDST, one-and-one-half times the expected rate in the general child population. Fifteen percent of the children failed one section on the DDST. Language was the most common area of delay (13%) followed by fine motor coordination (11%), gross motor coordination (6%), and personal-social skills (5%).

The school-aged homeless children frequently demonstrated academic difficulty. Almost one third of the school-aged children had repeated a grade (see Table 14.7). Homeless children often missed school. One half missed more than 1 week and one fifth missed more

Table 14.6 Percentage of Homeless Children With Reported Illness Symptoms Over Last Month

Symptom	Homeless (%) (N = 194)
Fever	38
Cough or cold	70
Vomiting or diarrhea	34
Ear infection	13
Sore throat with fever	15
Rash	15
Bronchitis or wheezing	10

than 3 weeks in the past 3 months. Among homeless children who were frequently absent, almost one half (16 of 33) missed school because their families were in transition.

HEALTH EVALUATION OF THE HOMELESS FAMILY

In evaluating the health of the homeless family, the health care professional must take into consideration the special characteristics and needs of this population. Additionally, once homeless, the family must focus its concerns on day-to-day survival and protection from external threats. The parents are frequently struggling to provide food, shelter, and other necessities for themselves and their children. As a result, parents may neglect their children's needs (such as emotional support, discipline, health care) that would, in securer family stituations, be considered essential. Because of this, homeless parents often feel guilty and have a sense of failure. Though the parents' initial attitude may be depressed, arrogant, demanding, or hostile, the practitioner should focus on helping the parent to feel accepted and to openly discuss family needs.

SUBJECTIVE DATA

A comprehensive health history on the child and family begins by the clinician asking the parent to describe his or her reason for coming to the clinic. During the initial visit with a homeless family, we recommend a brief but comprehensive, history that includes

Table 14.7 Percentage of Homeless Children With Grade Failure, Special Class Placement, and Excessive School Absenteeism

Item	Homeless (%) (N = 78)
Repeated a grade	30
Placed in special classes	28
Missed more than 1 week of school in past 3 months	42
Missed more than 3 weeks of school in past 3 months	17

preventive health care, development, school progress, and past medical history. The clinician should also inquire about the family's ability to meet basic needs of shelter, food, clothing, and security. Where have they been staying? With whom? What kind of situation is it? Why did they leave? What are their plans. How can you contact them for follow-up? Do they need assistance? The clinic must have sufficient referral resources to address basic needs such as food and housing. Unless these needs are met, the parent may find it difficult to attend to the health problems of the child.

Preventive Health Care

Homeless children and families are seldom current on routine preventive services such as a physical examination, and screening for anemia, vision, and hearing. If the parents are unsure when the child received these services, perform all preventive services to bring the child up to date. Homeless children are also at high risk for inadequate nutritional intake, failure to thrive, delayed growth, or obesity; therefore, each child's height and weight (and head circumference for children under 2 years of age) should be plotted.

Immunizations are usually not current, and the records have often been either lost or stolen. School enrollment can be delayed for weeks for lack of immunization documentation. Actively immunize children and reopen immunization records. The HIB (Haemophilus Influenza B), DPT (Diptheria, Pertusis, Tetanus), OPV (Polio), and MMR (Measles, Mumps, Rubella) vaccines are given according to the routine guidelines of the American Academy of Pediatrics (Committee on Infectious Disease, 1988). The most recent recommendations are to give an MMR at 12 months of age, and between 5 and 10 years of age. All children and adults born after 1956 should receive a second MMR vaccination. Because homeless children are a high-risk group for tuberculosis, they require a PPD annually. All black children should have a sickle cell screening test, which can be done as early as birth. Finally, children with a history of pica or anemia should have an free erythrocyte pretoporhorin to screen for lead exposure.

Development

Because of the high rate of developmental problems in homeless children, clinicians should perform a brief development screening on all children. This evaluation may include the parent self-administered Denver Pre-screening Development Questionnaire or an abbreviated administration of the DDST (Frankenberg et al., 1986). All children who fail the DDST should be referred to a local Regional Center for the Developmentally Disabled, where a comprehensive developmental evaluation can be performed.

The following case study provides an example of how referrals to agencies working with developmentally disabled children can make a difference in the lives of homeless children.

> In our outreach clinic, I saw a 13-month-old girl who had been a 1200-g premature infant. The mother's chief complaint was that the child had a cold. The infant was below the 5th percentile in growth, adjusted for her 12 weeks of prematurity. She had received no nutritional assessments, physical examinations, or immunizations since coming out of the hospital. Her age-adjusted development was normal. In addition to treating the cold, the health team gave immunizations and made referral to a "Failure to Thrive" Clinic at a local hospital for evaluation. In this clinic, the mother received intensive counseling on the nutritional needs of the infant and close monitoring of the infant's growth and development. We have continued to case manage the family, ensuring their continued attendance at the clinic, and we provide them with well child and episodic sick care. As a result, the mother was provided a more appropriate diet for the child, who is now growing at a more normal rate.

School Problems

Homeless children experience high rates of absenteeism and school failure. Therefore, it is also important to inquire about school enrollment, achievement, and homework problems. If there is any indication of academic difficulty, encourage the parents to seek an evaluation by the school of the child's progress. Because of the families' transience, schools often miss children with special needs; these children then do not receive the appropriate remedial service they are entitled to under the law. A note from the health provider is a powerful stimulus to the school system to perform academic testing and provide needed services to this population.

The Venice Family Clinic has developed a close working relationship with the two elementary schools where the local Westside Los Angeles shelters send their children. The clinic manager communicates frequently with the schools' principals, psychologists, and counselors. They respond rapidly to our requests for educational testing. The schools and clinic cooperate to resolve family problems that impact on the children (such as poor parental function owing to drug abuse). We have occasionally held a joint case conference for families with difficult problems.

The relationship is also beneficial to the schools. The clinic provides health screening, immunization, and other health services to homeless pupils referred to it by the schools. It also keeps the schools informed of health problems in the shelters. Health providers are available to school personnel by telephone. The relationship between the schools and the clinic has enabled homeless students to gain more rapid entry into school, miss less school, and obtain more timely comprehensive health and educational assessments.

Past Medical Problems

Because of the stresses of their daily lives and the constant struggle with the necessities of life, homeless families may neglect important health needs in their children. When they do come to a medical provider, their primary concerns are usually limited to the present, acute illness symptoms. Serious medical conditions may not be mentioned by the parent without prompting by the practitioner.

Therefore, a thorough inquiry into the child's past medical problems is very important. Use a quick, symptom-oriented "review of systems" to jog the parent's memory and improve the reporting of important past medical problems. A "review of systems" approach will often uncover specific medical symptoms that should be pursued in a diagnostic work-up.

Among homeless children, clinicians have found higher than expected incidences of asthma, anemia, cerebral palsy, seizure disorders, enuresis, encopresis, urinary tract infections, and other chronic health problems (Wood, Hayashi, Schossman, et al., 1989); Wright & Weber, 1987). Because the homeless family has often had poor access to medical care, these problems may not have been previously diagnosed.

Child Abuse Screening

Homeless families experience many problems that predispose them to child abuse, such as extreme family stress, exposure of the child to multiple caretakers, violence in the family and drug or alcohol abuse. Therefore, clinicians should screen for child abuse (neglect, physical and sexual) in the history and physical examination of every child.

Ask the parent(s) directly whether all the children are currently living with the family. If not, inquire where they are and whether the Department of Children's Protective Services has ever removed children from the family's custody. If the parents have a previous report for child abuse, obtain details about the dates the reports were made, their case worker's name, the type of abuse committed, the history of therapeutic intervention, and case disposition.

The behavior of the children is an excellent barometer for family stress in general and level of family functioning in particular. Ask the mother about, and observe the children for, destructive behavior, withdrawal, depression, anxiety, regressive behavior (such as bed-wetting in a previously toilet-trained child), or more profoundly disturbed behavior (such as rocking or self-mutilation). These may be signs of ongoing, unreported abuse or neglect.

Also, carefully observe the mother for signs of current drug or alcohol intoxication, or signs of previous drug or alcohol abuse. Do a detailed drug and alcohol use history if there is any suspicion of a problem. Inquiries of this type are seldom answered honestly, but they can give the clinician a sense of existing substance abuse.

If the clinician is suspicious of drug or alcohol abuse in the parent, or is unsure about the existence of child abuse or neglect, the public health outreach team should be notified to work closely with the parents and continue the family observation. If child abuse or neglect is suspected, then it must be reported immediately to the Department of Children's Services.

OBJECTIVE DATA

Objective information is gained when first interacting with the mother: observe her affect and speech for signs of depression, anger, confusion, ambivalence, or more profound mental illness. Signs in the mother such as extreme hostility or suspicion, indifference toward the child's health, or abnormally low body weight, may be signs of drug abuse in the family. Note the interaction of the family as a unit—the amount of communication, expression of affection, discipline, and organization.

It is important to be sensitive to the maturity level of the children's behavior. Homeless children often display "pseudomature" behavior that appears mature on the surface but may be actually maladaptive. For example, 3-year-old children may be immediately affectionate with strange adults of whom they should be initially suspicious. A 4-year-old may act as the part-time caretaker for a year-old sibling, performing duties such as diapering or feeding. These may be signs of extreme stress on the child and family, and call for further evaluation by a mental health professional.

The following case study exemplifies how families under extreme stress may present to the clinician.

> A mother brought her 2-year-old to see me because she had a fever. On the physical examination, the child had otitis media and no other medical problems. The medical history revealed that the child was behind in her immunizations and had not seen a doctor for more than a year, despite the fact that she had been a premature infant who was treated for 6 months with phenobarbitol for neonatal seizures. The mother did not know why the medication had been stopped. More importantly, during the interaction, the mother appeared distracted, aloof, and irritable. She was very short-tempered with the child, who was very aggressive and difficult to control. In a clinical team meeting, we discussed the mother and child, and decided to follow the family closely in coordination with the public health nurse. During the next few weeks, we received several reports that the mother seemed intoxicated at times and used particularly severe punishment on her child. It became apparent that the mother was addicted to cocaine. Three weeks after we began following the family closely, the mother, while on a drug binge, left her child alone for more than 24 hours. She was reported to the Department of Children's Services, and the child was removed from her care.

Physical Examination

As noted earlier, the child's initial complaint may not be the most serious medical problem. It is common for a history or physical examination to uncover serious disorders in a homeless child presenting with only minor complaints. In addition to treating the child for the initial complaint, the clinician should also search for other acute problems that are common in homeless children. These conditions include ear infections, colds, tooth decay and tooth infections, lice or scabies, conjunctivitis, allergies, skin infections, diaper rashes, cuts, abrasions, bruises, and broken bones.

The physical examination should also include a careful inspection for the following chronic problems: visual acuity or strabismus, sinus infections with chronic nasal congestion and purulent nasal discharge, hearing problems, heart murmurs, anemia, asthma or bronchitis, constipation and encopresis, eczema, and neurological signs such as weakness, asymmetry, or spasticity.

If there is sufficient privacy, every physical examination should include a genital examination for signs of sexual abuse. The skin and extremities should also be carefully inspected for new or old traumatic injury. Explanations by the parents should be explored. Any questionable or suspicious findings should be first reported to the Department of Children's Protective Services and then referred to a specialist for further examination and an in-depth interview with the family. It is important to report suspicious cases immediately because homeless families may move away or purposefully flee before a more extensive evaluation for child abuse can be conducted.

Laboratory

On the initial visit, we recommend the following laboratory examinations be performed according to the recommendations of the American Academy of Pediatrics (1988): screening for anemia, vision and hearing, and a urinalysis. If the child presents with diarrhea, a stool culture is recommended. There have been several outbreaks of shigella in the shelters we serve, and the stool culture is used as much for epidemiological surveillance and disease control as for clinical management.

ASSESSMENT AND PLAN

An effective health plan for homeless children requires the clinic to develop an extensive outreach and follow-up system. This outreach system should include an outreach team, minimally consisting of a public health nurse and a community worker (See chapter 3 by Cousineau, Casanova, and Erlenbusch on case management). Table 14.8 lists the responsibilities of the nurse and community worker in the outreach team.

The outreach team assists families to follow medical regimens and to accept services such as psychiatric counseling, parenting classes, and follow-up health visits. The outreach team will be better able than the clinic team to help the family set priorities and help them incorporate the clinical recommendations into their life in the shel-

Table 14.8 Responsibilities of Outreach Practitioner and Family Case Manager

Outreach public health nurse:
Develop and maintain trusting relationship with families
Follow up acutely ill family members
   Review medicines and treatment plans
   Facilitate referrals and follow up on referrals
   Provide feedback to health care teams
Perform field assessments and triage to clinic
Provide health education and disease prevention
Continue assessment and follow-up for child abuse-neglect in high-risk families
Family case manager:
Develop and maintain trusting relationship with families
Help family set priorities and develop goals to meet them (e.g., find housing, resolve relationship problems, drug rehabilitation, find job, etc.)
Assist families in progress toward meeting goals
Provide family advocacy with public agencies (welfare, WIC, housing authority, etc.)
Provide family advocacy with health agencies

ter. Families in such stressful living conditions and with such a wide array of problems need an advocate outside the clinic who can see their whole situation, follow up on problems, and help the family develop priorities to address their health as well as other basic needs.

CASE STUDY

The following case study is used to illustrate the comprehensive approach we feel is indicated for homeless families. The case was chosen to be representative of the types of problems we see and their degree of complexity.

Subjective Data

The mother's chief concern is that her 8-month-old boy has diarrhea. The diarrhea occurs four times a day and fills the diaper. There is no blood in the stool, vomiting, fever, or rash. The child is mildly irritable but taking fluids well. The review of his past medical history reveals that he was under 5 pounds at birth and remained in the hospital 1 month. He was hospitalized at 2 months of age for a fever. The mother is not quite sure what he had, but he was in the hospital 10 days. The review of systems does not reveal any other problems. The child is behind on his immunizations and has had only one well-child health visit in his life. By a quick developmental history, it appears the child may be delayed; he cannot sit alone. His social skills and upper extremity motor skills appear normal by history. The mother is not with an adult partner, and she has no other children. The mother became homeless because she was recently dropped from welfare for reasons unclear to her. She has no money, food, or plans for shelter for the night. She has been living in a male friend's car, but she does not want to go back to that situation because she feels it is dangerous.

Objective Data

The mother is moderately hostile and appears detached and depressed. On physical examination of the child, he is afebrile, well hydrated, and active, and his growth parameters are tenth percentile for his age. The physical examination is normal except that the neurological examination shows mild hypertonicity in the lower extremities, and he is unstable in the sitting position. He has a normal grasp and passes objects hand to hand. On a full Denver Developmental Screening Test, he fails the gross motor section and passes the fine motor, personal-social, and language section. A screening hematocrit is 30%. Table 14.9 presents a sample assessment and plan for this case.

CONCLUSION

Often the number and complexity of health problems in a homeless family are overwhelming for the clinician as well as for the family. When a clinic-based team and an outreach team work together, it becomes a powerful intervention in the lives of homeless families. Social and medical problems that would only frustrate the clinic-based practitioner are responsive to a coordinated approach with an outreach team. Under this case management approach, many of our homeless families at the Venice Family Clinic have responded quite well. They begin to develop a new self-confidence and to take control of their children's health and their own lives. It is rewarding to address complex psychosocial and physical health needs of a family and see the healing, growth, and progress that may result.

Table 14.9 Case Study Assessment and Plan

Problem	Assessment	Plan
1	Housing, safety, food, transportation—family has no place to stay, needs clothes and help requalifying for welfare or looking for a job	Emergency housing voucher or same-day referral to a shelter; referral to outreach team for welfare advocacy, food pantry, clothes distribution agency referral Bus tokens for transportation Close follow-up by outreach team case manager
2	Diarrhea—child's diarrhea appears mild with no dehydration or fever	Stool culture for surveillance Oral rehydration fluid information and education on transition diet, give 2-day supply of soy formula Refer to outreach nurse for next-day follow-up evaluation and education; notify public health nurse of pending culture
3	Questionable developmental delay	Refer to the regional center for complete evaluation; outreach team should encourage the mother to follow through and check on compliance with appointments
4	Anemia	Give the mother education on iron-containing foods and a WIC referral; notify public health nurse of referral Treat with ferrous sulfate at 3 to 5 mg of elemental iron of body weight
5	Well child care—immunizations, nutrition, growth	Give immunizations during this visit despite the mild illness
6	Question of maternal depression	Refer mother to local mental health agency in coordination with outreach team

REFERENCES

American Academy of Pediatrics. (1988). Guidelines for Health Supervision II. Elk Grove, IL: American Academy of Pediatrics.

———. Report on the Committee on Infectious Diseases. Elk Grove, IL: American Academy of Pediatrics.

Frankenburg, W. K., et al. (1983). The Denver pre-screening developmental questionnaire (PDQ). *Pediatrics, 57,* 744–753.

Hartman, C. (1983). *America's housing crisis: What is to be done?* Boston: Routledge and Kegan.

Jaffe, M., Harel, J., Goldberg, A., et al. (1980). The use of the Denver developmental screening test in infant welfare clinics. *Developmental Medicine and Child Neurology, 22,* 55–60.

Mak, H., Johnston, P., Abbey, H., et al. (1982). Prevalence of asthma and health service utilization of asthmatic children in an inner city. *Journal of Allergy Clinical Immunology, 70,* 367–372.

New York Coalition for the Homeless. (1986). *Hungry children and Mr. Cuomo: Time for Action.* New York: Author.

Siegel, S., & Rachelefsky, G. (1986). Asthma in infants and children: I. *Journal of Allergy Clinical Immunology, 76*(1), 1–14.

U. S. Conference of Mayors. (1984). *Homeless in America.* Washington, DC: Government Printing Office.

U. S. Conference of Mayors. (1986). *The continued growth of hungry homelessness and poverty in America's cities.* Washington, DC: Government Printing Office.

U. S. Congress, House of Representatives. (1986). *Safety net programs: Are they reaching children* [Hearings Before the Select Committee on Children, Youth and Families]? Washington, DC: Government Printing Office.

Wood, D., Hayashi, T., Schossman, S., et al. (1989). *Over the brink: Homeless families in Los Angeles.* Sacramento: California Assembly Office of Research.

Wood, D., Valdez, R. B., Hayashi, T., et al. *The health of homeless children: A comparison study.* Pediatrics 1990; 86:858–866.

Wright, J. D., & Weber, E. (1987). *Homelessness and health.* New York: McGraw-Hill.

Mental Health Issues

Medical Care of Homeless and Runaway Adolescents

15

Jennifer R. Garshman, Charlene G. Sand-
ers, Gary L. Yates, Richard G. MacKenzie

CHAPTER HIGHLIGHTS

- The Department of Health and Human Services estimates the national number of homeless and runaway youth to be as many as one million, of which approximately one-quarter million become "permanently" homeless.
- Adolescents usually become homeless because they have run away from, or been thrown out of, dysfunctional family units where physical and sexual abuse is common.
- Homelessness places extreme stress on the adolescent during an already tumultuous period of change, development and personality formation.
- Homeless adolescents are usually school drop-outs with no previous work history and few job skills. They commonly rely on illicit activities for survival such as prostitution, pornography, drug-dealing and petty theft.
- The vast majority of homeless adolescents have serious health problems such as severe depression with suicidal ideation, pregnancy, drug abuse and multiple sexually transmitted diseases.
- The homeless adolescent is at exceptionally high risk for HIV infection. A 1988 Covenant House study of 16 to 21 year old runaways in New York demonstrated a HIV infection rate of 6%.
- The evaluation of a homeless adolescent should be guided by the HEADS psychosocial profile (an acronym for Home, Education, Activities/Affect, Drug use, and Sex/Suicide/Satanic abuse).

215

- Maximal treatment should be initiated for all conditions diagnosed at the first encounter because the homeless adolescent may never return to the clinic.
- Medical-legal policies surrounding the treatment of homeless youths are often fraught with confusion, due to the complexity of and geographic variations in minors' consent laws.

INTRODUCTION

Homeless and runaway adolescents are a rapidly growing segment of the homeless population. The Department of Health and Human Services estimates the national number of homeless and runaway youth to be as many as one million, of which approximately one-quarter million become "permanently" homeless (U.S. Department of Health and Human Services, 1983).

Adolescents become homeless for different reasons from their adult and young child counterparts. As a rule, they are not homeless because of economic hardship. Instead, they have run away from, or been thrown out of, dysfunctional family units or broken homes where physical and sexual abuse is common. As a result, most homeless adolescents are runaways or throwaways, disenfranchised from their biological families.

Data from the Childrens Hospital of Los Angeles High Risk Youth Program in 1985 showed that more than one third of runaway adolescents had experienced physical and sexual abuse, as compared with only 7% of nonrunaways (Yates, MacKenzie, Pennbridge, & Cohen, 1988). In such cases, the act of running away may be viewed as an adaptive behavior; it is actually a solution. Family reunification is rarely a viable option.

Once homeless, they use different survival adaptations as well. It is these differences that influence the spectrum of health problems seen in adolescents and influence the way in which they interact with the medical system. Such youngsters find themselves alone on the streets without adult supervision or guidance, but lacking sufficient maturity to protect themselves. They recreate "families" on the streets by banding together into peer groups, or by attaching to older pimps for protection and support. Runaway youths have often been victimized by adults, both at home and on the streets, and are distrustful of authority figures including health providers and social workers. This presents a barrier to care because they often will not be trusting enough to seek medical care until they are truly desperate with an advanced medical problem.

Runaway adolescents are usually school dropouts with no previous work history and few if any legal marketable job skills. Commonly, they must rely on illicit activities for survival such as prostitution, pornography, drug dealing, and petty theft. Additionally, many youth find it necessary to trade sex for food, shelter, or protection—so-called survival sex. Such adolescents are at increased risk for assault, rape, emotional trauma, unwanted pregnancies, and STDs including HIV disease.

Adolescence itself is a complicating factor. Adolescence has been described as a period of turbulent change stemming from biological growth and psychological maturation. Normative behavior during these years involves experimentation, testing of physical and emotional limits, and exploration of sexuality and peer group relationships. For adolescents in relatively stable, nurturing environments these "wonder years" can be trying even with the benefit of family support and activity. Homeless youth must master these adolescent developmental milestones with the meager and deviant resources of the streets. Without adult support, these normal developmental tasks can be taken to very risky extremes.

COMMON MEDICAL DIAGNOSES

Table 15.1 provides an overview of the frequency of medical diagnoses of runaway adolescents at their first clinic visit at the Los Angeles Free Clinic in 1985 (Yates et al. 1988). It demonstrates that most health problems are a direct consequence of street life and of those adaptations required to survive.

Mental health problems such as depression and suicidal ideation are startlingly common. Eighty-four percent of the adolescents seen in the clinic were judged to be clinically depressed, with fully 9% being actively suicidal. Runaway adolescents frequently feel trapped, unable to return home to their dysfunctional families, yet unable to nurture themselves because they lack stable financial and emotional resources. They frequently carry with them the emotional scars of past physical and sexual abuse.

Some form of drug use was reported by 84% of runaway adolescents. Drug abuse was seen in more than one half of the youth, with intravenous drug use noted in more than one third. Drugs are used to

Table 15.1 Medical Diagnoses of Homeless Adolescents and Runaways

	Frequency	
Diagnoses	(%)	(%)
Mental health disturbance		93
Depression	84	
Actively suicidal		89
Drug use overall	84	
Drug abuse		57
Intravenous drug use	35	
Diagnosis-related sexual activity		55
Family planning/abortion	20	
STDs	18	
Pregnancy	13	
Pelvic inflammatory disease	4	
Physical vulnerability		6
Trauma	4	
Rape		2
Medical		19
Pneumonia	8	
Scabies	6	
Hepatitis	3	
Asthma	2	

Note. Adapted from "A Risk Profile Comparison of Runaway and Non-Runaway Youth" by G. Yates, R. MacKenzie, J. Pennbridge, and E. Cohen, 1988, *American Journal of Public Health*, 78, pp. 820–821. Copyright © 1988 by Yates. Adapted by permission. Multiple diagnoses per patient was allowed; therefore percentages total more than 100%.

self-medicate depression or other mental health disorders, to remain awake at night to "turn tricks," to relieve boredom, or just to have fun.

The consequences of sexual activity were diagnosed in more than one half of the adolescents' visits: pregnancy, and pregnancy-related morbidity and STDs including pelvic inflammatory disease. HIV seropositivity has been seen at increasingly high rates among runaway adolescents because of prostitution and intravenous drug use. A 1988 Covenant House study of runaways in New York demonstrated a HIV positivity rate in 16- to 21-year-olds of 6% (Kennedy, 1988). Our own tracking of HIV seriologies at the Children's Hospital Adolescent Clinic in 1989 showed a 2% HIV seropositive rate among 12 to 24-year-olds, which included many runaways.

Physical vulnerability, manifested by the diagnoses of trauma and rape, was noted in 6%. Purely medical complaints such as respiratory and skin problems constituted only 19% of total diagnoses.

PSYCHOSOCIAL PROFILE

It becomes obvious that significant morbidity in the homeless adolescent population is due to life-style and that directing attention only to purely medical complaints is inadequate. Therefore, an in-depth psychosocial evaluation is a crucial part of medical care. The psychosocial interview used by the Children's Hospital of Los Angeles High Risk Youth Program is the home, education, activities-affect, drug use, sex-suicide-satanic abuse (HEADS) profile (see Table 15.2). A psychosocial interview covering these topics provides a quick "biopsy slice" of the adolescent's psychosocial being. This profile of

Table 15.2 Heads Psychological Profile

H—Home	Living where now?
	Why and when left home (abuse)?
	What is present relationship with family members?
E—Education	Level completed
	Goals
A—Activities	Friends?
	Pleasurable activities
	How does patient support self?
	Aspirations
	Affect
D—Drugs	Type, route, amount
	How paid for (trading sex for drugs)?
	Does patient view use as a problem?
	Is rehabilitation desired?
S—Sex	Orientation
	Estimated number of partners (male, female)
	Contraception
	Previous STDs, previous pregnancies
	Condom use
	Survival sex
—Suicide	Current ideation; if yes, assess risk
	Past attempts; if yes, describe number,
	Method, precipitant
—Satanic abuse	Cult involvement?

questions should be asked by the medical provider during the initial encounter and is updated briefly in an abbreviated form at each subsequent visit. It is designed to progress from least threatening to most sensitive subject matter as the interview proceeds.

The home portion of this profile is used to define the adolescent's current living situation. Is it satisfactory and safe? Does the adolescent want shelter placement? Also, it is important to investigate why the youth left home and search for evidence of abuse to evaluate the potential for reunification with family.

The Activities section is helpful to gain a sense of how the adolescent interacts in a social setting. Is he or she able to establish peer relationships? An effective approach is to ask if he or she has a best friend. Additionally, it is crucial to ascertain how an adolescent is supporting himself or herself. Is survival sex involved?

The questions in the drug section assess for substance abuse and, if appropriate, for the adolescent's readiness for drug rehabilitation. Does the youth view the drug use as a problem?

The series of questions in the sex segment of HEADS evaluate for sexual healthiness and safety. Are contraception and condoms being used? Is there a history of sexual abuse or a need for survival sex? Adolescence is the time to explore and define sexuality. Through questioning one must make sure this process is happening as smoothly as possible.

In the suicide portion, ask directly about suicidal ideation and assess the seriousness of the risk of suicide. Satanic abuse is included in the profile because these behaviors are increasingly common. These behaviors are an urgent cry for help on the part of the adolescent and usually require a special set of referrals and levels of support (such as clergy involvement).

Numerous social and psychological problems will likely be uncovered during this interview process. To address these issues adequately, a health team should include medical personnel, social workers, and mental health providers working in concert to address simultaneously the health along with primary survival needs of food, shelter, clothes, and income. Addressing simply the medical complaint while ignoring the social environment is tantamount to covering a gaping wound with a Band-Aid. For example, an adolescent cannot decrease his or her HIV risk from prostitution until he or she has found an alternative way to get money for food and shelter.

Anticipatory guidance about sexual activity and choices, STDs, HIV, contraception, nutrition, and substance abuse should be offered to all adolescents. In female adolescents, the history should include the date of the last normal menstrual period. Runaway adolescents are usually unable to contribute details of past medical history or of family history.

MEDICAL EXAMINATION

The usual principles of well-adolescent care should be applied to the homeless adolescent, with additional attention to those illnesses for which the homeless are at increased risk. All adolescents need a complete health evaluation at least once during the adolescent years to assess for proper physical and behavioral growth. Optimally, a comprehensive evaluation is recommended every 2 years to assess the risk profile, provide anticipatory guidance, and assess the progression of pubescence. Runaway adolescents, coming usually from dysfunctional families, have often received inadequate health care in the past, even while at home.

Particularly important aspects of the physical examination include the following:

1. Assessment for proper growth and development including sexual maturation.
2. Examination of breasts and testes; instruction in self-examination. Testicular cancer, albeit rare, is the most common solid tumor in males under 30 years of age (Neinstein, 1984).
3. Screening for STDs and pregnancy (see later section for more details). Assume that all runaways are at risk for complications of sexual activity. In all asymptomatic adolescents, screen for chlamydia and syphilis at least annually. In asymptomatic female adolescents, screen also for gonorrhea and cervical dysplasia because of the widespread prevalence of human papilloma virus. Repeat syphilis serologies whenever any new STD is diagnosed. Consider HIV testing.
4. A hematocrit. Anemia is common during adolescence because of rapid growth and of menstrual loss in female adolescents. In the runaway, this is compounded by malnutrition.
5. Perform a dipstick urinalysis for nitrites, white blood cells, protein, and glucose to assess for occult renal disease, urinary tract infections, and diabetes.

6. Give all immunizations to bring the adolescent up to date including the following:
    (a) dT (diptheria, tetanus) (every 10 years)
    (b) MMR (should avoid during pregnancy; perform a urine B-HCG first); Also, avoid giving MMR the 3 months preceding conception, although this is very impractical)
    (c) PPD (every 1 to 2 years in this population)

PRINCIPLES OF CARE

There are several principles that are central to the history, physical, and ongoing clinical relationship with a homeless and runaway adolescent: maintain confidentiality, have a nonjudgmental approach, provide maximal therapy at each visit, always assess for suicide potential, and work with other agencies to provide care.

Adolescents are frequently suspicious of adults asking personal questions such as those contained in the HEADS psychosocial interview. Adolescents need to be reassured of the confidential nature of the doctor-patient relationship. Note that many of the questions posed could incriminate the youth in illegal activity like prostitution and drug dealing. There are limits to this confidentiality; child abuse and active suicidal or homicidal ideation by law cannot be kept secret. Patients should be made aware of these limits at the start of the encounter.

Runaway adolescents are often forced by circumstances into activities that they find embarrassing or humiliating. They may also be exploring sexual roles with which they are not yet comfortable. Allowing the adolescent to disclose these activities in a safe, nonjudgmental environment enhances the accuracy of the medical history and encourages trust and compliance with medical regimens.

The homeless adolescent may never return to the clinic for a second or subsequent visit, regardless of the nature of their medical or social problems. Consequently, maximal medical treatment should be given initially. For example, a youth with an exudative pharyngitis should be treated empirically for streptococcal disease. A homeless female adolescent with a vaginal discharge showing greater than 10 to 20 white blood cells per high-power field should be treated presumptively for chlamydia and gonococcal cervicitis while cultures are pending. Presumptive treatment should be adopted whenever public health prevention and cost-effectiveness are considerations.

Evaluate for active suicidal ideation at each visit. As was previously described, 9% of runaway adolescents at their first clinical encounter were actively suicidal in the Los Angeles study. If as a clinician you are not comfortable with this assessment it is important to work with a social worker or psychologist who can make these assessments.

Networking of medical and social service providers serving runaway adolescents in a particular community maximizes services for the youth and eliminates duplication of work for staff. The homeless outreach clinic that serves adolescents should have close working relationships with Travelers Aid, youth hostels and shelters, local food pantries, the schools and adult education organizations, the public health department, and a local hospital.

SEXUALLY TRANSMITTED DISEASES AND SEXUAL ASSAULT

STDs are endemic to homeless adolescent groups. Sexual activity with multiple, often anonymous, partners is the norm because many adolescents must barter sex for shelter and food. Consequently, it is essential to search for signs of STDs regardless of the presenting complaint and to screen asymptomatic youth periodically as well.

The most common STDs in the adolescent population are human papilloma virus and chlamydia. Human papilloma virus infections most frequently present as genital warts, but may also result in cervical dysplasia accounting for the increasing rate of abnormal Pap smears in young female adolescents. Chlamydia may be asymptomatic in both male and female adolescents, or may cause symptomatic cervicitis, urethritis, dysuria, pelvic inflammatory disease, and epididymitis. Homeless youngsters often delay seeking medical treatment until forced by advanced complications such as the pain of pelvic inflammatory disease. Also prevalent are gonorrhea, herpes simplex virus, pubic lice, genital scabies, syphilis, and vaginitis such as Candida, trichomonas, and bacterial vaginosis.

We recommend that all asymptomatic, sexually active adolescents should have syphilis and chlamydia testing annually. Asymptomatic, sexually active female adolescents should also have gonorrhea testing and a Pap smear annually. A male adolescent requires directed STD evaluation if he has a urethral discharge, dysuria, anal discharge, anal pain, or anogenital lesions. The female adolescent requires STD-directed evaluation if she presents with vaginal discharge, unexplained lower abdominal pain, unexplained dysuria, abnormal vaginal bleeding, anal pain, anal discharge, or anogenital lesions.

STDs frequently coexist. Therefore, any youth with symptoms consistent with any STD should be evaluated for chlamydia, gonorrhea, and syphilis. HIV testing may be considered. Risk factors for HIV, such as intravenous drug use, unprotected sex and sex with unknown partners should be assessed. The diagnosis of a new STD may be used as an opportunity to reinforce safer-sex practices. Empirical treatment is usually advised because youths may not return to the clinic for diagnostic confirmation and treatment.

Sexual victimization is customary in street life. For adolescents relying on sexual activity for survival, the line between consent and coercion is grossly blurred. Many youths view sex as the currency with which they barter for shelter, food, and drugs. Adolescents experiencing sexual harassment and violence are hesitant to identify assailants, as these same individuals may at other times be protectors and survival "resources." Often, the psychological markers of sexual assault are more visible than the physical abnormalities, such as depressed mood, nonspecific anxiety, a detached or "I don't care" attitude.

Medical evaluation for a sexually assaulted adolescent should include a urine pregnancy test, screening for gonorrhea and chlamydia in all sites used in sexual intercourse (mouth, anus, vagina), and a syphilis serology. HIV testing should also be considered. If the assault is recent, the adolescent should be treated empirically with ceftriaxone for gonorrhea and chlamydia. If the assault occurred within 72 hours prior to the exam the female adolescent should be offered pregnancy prophylaxis. This is accomplished with two Ovral tablets at once and again in 12 hours (Neinstein, 1984). Care of these abused youngsters should be nonpunitive, and treatment should be reinforced with supportive services.

PREGNANCY

Homeless female adolescents are at high risk for becoming pregnant. In many cases, the pregnancy is unexpected and unwanted, or there is significant ambivalence. Homeless adolescents have inadequate access to contraception and limited support for compliance if contraception is available. If the pregnancy is planned, it is often undertaken with the mistaken feeling that it will provide for their unmet emotional needs of love and security.

Should a homeless adolescent decide to continue a pregnancy to term, both she and the developing infant face health consequences by virtue of maternal young age and by her state of homelessness. Anemia, toxemia, and maternal mortality rates are increased in pregnant adolescents when compared with counterparts in their 20s (Neinstein, 1984). Among homeless adolescents, their baseline health is often poor and is made worse by pregnancy, and further impaired by inconsistent and inadequate nutrition. Access to early and consistent prenatal care is crucial but often very difficult to obtain because of lack of resources and reluctance on the part of the adolescent to seek care.

Infants born to homeless adolescents are susceptible to the mother's high-risk life-style. Drugs, exposure to physical violence, and sexual promiscuity with its threat of HIV and syphilis pose a health risk to the developing fetus and later to the infant. Moreover, runaway youths, having no role models for healthy parenting, are likely to possess suboptimal parenting skills unless strong social support is provided.

The medical evaluation of the pregnant adolescent includes a complete physical examination to assess general health status and a pelvic examination to determine the correct age of the fetus and establish the expected arrival date. Laboratory evaluation needs to include a confirmatory b-HCG (urine or blood), hematocrit (owing to the high incidence of anemia), baseline rubella titer, syphilis serology, dipstick urinalysis, Pap smear, microscopic vaginal wet mount, and cervical cultures for gonorrhea and chlamydia, and, as now required by law, hepatitis B screening. HIV testing should be offered.

Nonjudgmental pregnancy counseling delineating possible options should be offered as soon as pregnancy is confirmed. These options include continuation of pregnancy, with the possibility of adoption, or pregnancy termination if the gestational date permits. A discussion of possible consequences of high-risk life-styles and improper nutrition is undertaken. Pregnant youth must be apprised of the potential danger HIV and drug use may have on fetal viability and neonatal health. Often, a desire for a healthy baby may be the impetus for change to a healthier life-style.

Each pregnancy embodies complex issues, and the ultimate outcome is frequently undecided at the end of the first visit. If ambivalent, the youth can be encouraged to continue the decision-making process during the next few days, and return for further counseling and support. Because a return visit can never be guaranteed, all appropriate referrals should be made during the first encounter, and prenatal vitamins should be dispensed.

HIV DISEASE

Runaway and homeless adolescents are at exceptional risk for HIV infection because of life-styles involving survival sex and substance abuse. HIV pretest counseling should be offered to any adolescent who requests testing and to any at-risk adolescent identified by staff. This counseling should be done by a skilled professional who can impart HIV education and can assess the youth's emotional readiness to receive positive or negative test results. As soon as the adolescent is felt to be emotionally and intellectually able to grasp the con- sequences of the test results, testing should occur. Posttest counseling needs to include a review of educational information taught during the first session, and appropriate referrals and support including dispensing of condoms and bleach. Patients are encouraged to enroll in drug rehabilitation programs. Referrals to shelters and to job- training programs, such as the Jobs Corps, decrease the dependence on survival sex. Adolescents who test negative are encouraged to return for repeat testing in 3 months and then again every 3 to 6 months while unsafe behavior continues. Those who test positive may need acute crisis intervention, and careful assessment for active suicidal ideation is essential. Referrals for suicide hotlines and emergency support services need to be made available. Lastly, the adolescent should be linked with a medical provider familiar with HIV disease.

Most HIV-positive adolescents have been recently infected through high-risk sexual or drug behavior. Because the estimated latency period is 7 to 10 years, most infected youth will not develop AIDS until early adulthood. Therefore, the primary goals in caring for adolescents are health maintenance, recognition of early immune deterioration, and prompt diagnosis and treatment of concurrent illnesses, such as syphilis and tuberculosis, which could hasten HIV progression. When absolute CD4 counts drop below 500, AZT therapy should be initiated as this has clearly been shown to slow progression of disease and improve quality of life (Katz, 1989). The asymptomatic adolescent is encouraged to receive medical screening every 3 to 6 months; the symptomatic adolescent needs attention more frequently. A discussion of the comprehensive HIV-directed history, review of systems, and physical examination is outlined in chapter 8 by Avery and O'Connell on HIV and homeless persons, much of which is applicable to adolescents.

SOCIAL SERVICES

Homeless adolescents roam urban streets and camp out in vacant buildings throughout the United States. They may be very far from familiar territory and unaware of how and where to ask for help. These youths exist in an isolated subculture out of the "mainstream," making it difficult for social service providers to access them. Frequently, a homeless adolescent may only interface with mainstream society when desperate for medical care. Consequently, the medical visit is crucial to play a role in linking the adolescent and youth-serving professionals. Model programs using street outreach workers and mobile health teams have attempted to reach out to adolescents on their own "turf." Such field professionals are more likely to establish trust and rapport. They make excellent allies and can provide competent health education, make referrals to the clinic, and assist clinicians with following up on adolescents' medical and psychosocial progress.

Runaway adolescents need extensive support to rejoin the mainstream. They will require extensive referrals for immediate shelter, food, and clothing. They will need job training, educational counseling, emotional support, and often drug rehabilitation. Maximal aid can be offered when a community's medical and other youth-serving agencies are closely aligned. This allows multiple professionals to work cooperatively, without duplicated effort for the benefit of a particular youngster.

LEGAL AND ETHICAL ISSUES

Medical-legal policies surrounding the treatment of runaway and homeless youths are often fraught with confusion. The dilemma stems from the currently perplexing state of minors' consent laws.

Unfortunately, these laws vary from one locale to another. Any youth-serving professional must have an understanding of their state's minors' consent laws and emancipated minor criteria.

Informed consent is the cornerstone of the implicit contractual agreement that typifies the health-provider-patient relationship. First, however, adolescents must be able to give an *informed* consent. It must be established that the adolescent (a) understands the nature of the therapy, and (b) appreciates the risks and benefits of the proposed treatment plan. In addition, it needs to be determined if harm to the adolescent will occur if treatment is delayed or prevented. Therapeutic modalities should be in the best interest of the adolescent (Rosoff, 1981). Medical team members are obligated to document the adolescent's ability to understand a proper informed consent.

All states have laws that regulate minors' access to reproductive health. Most states permit minors to consent to diagnosis and treatment of STDs and pregnancy, and to acquire contraception. Access to abortion varies greatly between states. Health care workers are strongly urged to investigate their local laws. Rules will vary according to patient's age, marital status, medical condition, financial status, and education level.

The most useful medical-legal concept for dealing with homeless adolescents is the use of emancipation criteria. Emancipation entitles adolescents to consent to all forms of health care, except sterilization, as if they were adults. There is state-to-state variation for the definition of an emancipated minor. An acceptable description of emancipation may include any of the following:

1. Persons of specific age (usually 18 years)
2. Minors who are or who have been married
3. Minors who are parents
4. Minors who are living away from home, managing their own finances
5. Minors in the armed forces
6. Minors who are high school graduates
7. Minors living at home, but working and contributing to their own support
8. Emancipation by court decree

An alternative mode of using minors' consent is via the "mature minor doctrine" (Hoffman & Greydanus, 1989). This form of minors' consent has enabled numerous adolescent advocate programs to carry out their counseling efforts. The doctrine places exclusive emphasis on cognitive competence, independent of age, residence, financial means, and parental wishes. The decision to provide care is based solely on the judgment of the medical practitioner that the adolescent is mature and competent.

In the ideal setting, minors' consent laws help homeless youth receive better health care. For adolescents caught on the streets, the ability to dictate their own medical well-being is crucial to survival and improves self-esteem. For disenfranchised, runaway youth, the act of self-consent may be the first step toward validation of self-importance.

CONCLUSION

Street youth are usually homeless because they are running away from an intolerable home situation. They are trying to survive and grow up in a harsh and frequently exploitative environment. Their survival adaptations may offer short-term solutions but often lead to serious health problems. Appropriate health care should target both medical and psychosocial concerns.

REFERENCES

American Academy of Pediatrics. (1988). *Red Book.* Elk Grove Village, IL: American Academy of Pediatrics.

Breakey, W. R., Fischer, P., Kramer, M., et al. (1989). Special communication: Health and mental health problems of homeless men and women in Baltimore. *Journal of the American Medical Association, 262,* 1351–1358.

Centers for Disease Control. (1987, June 5). Leads from the MMWR—Tuberculosis control among homeless populations. *Journal of the American Medical Association, 257,* 2886–2888.

Centers for Disease Control. (1989a, September 1). 1989 Sexually transmitted diseases treatment guidelines. *Morbidity and Mortality Weekly Report.*

Centers for Disease Control. (1989b, November). AIDS cases—Cumulative through October, 1989. *HIV/AIDS Surveillance, 10.*

Council on Scientific Affairs. (1989, September 8). Health care needs of homeless and runaway youths. *Journal of the American Medical Association, 262,* 1358–1361.

Goldenring, J. M., & Cohen, E. (1988, July). Getting into adolescent heads. *Contemporary Pediatrics, 5,* 75–90.

Hofmann, A., & Greydanus, D. (Eds.). (1989). *Adolescent medicine* (2nd ed.). Norwalk, CT: Appleton and Lange.

Institute of Medicine, Committee on Health for Homeless People. (1988). *Homelessness, health, and human needs.* Washington, DC: National Academy Press.

Katz, M. (1989, October). *Unpublished data from the AIDS Clinical Trial Group—019.* Presented at The National Aids Update, San Francisco.

Kennedy, J. (1988). *Convenant House study.* Unpublished data, New York.

Morrissey, J., Hofman, A., & Thrope, J. (1986). *Consent and confidentiality in the health care of children and adolescents: A legal guide.* New York: Free Press.

Neinstein, L. (1984). *Adolescent health care: A practical guide.* Baltimore: Urban and Schwarzenberg.

Phair, J., et al. (1990, January 18). The risk of *Pneumocyctis carinii* pneumonia among men infected with human immunodeficiency virus, type I. *New England Journal of Medicine, 322,* 161–165.

Robertson, M., & Cousineau, M. (1986). Health status and access to health services among the urban homeless. *American Journal of Public Health, 76,* 561–563.

Rosoff, A. (1981). *Informed consent: A guide for health care providers.* Rockville, MD: Aspen.

Shaffer, D., & Canton, C. (1984). *Runaway and homeless youth in New York City.* Report to the Ittleson Foundation. New York: Columbia University College of Physicians and Surgeons.

U.S. Department of Health and Human Services. (1983, October). *Runaway and Homeless Youth.* Washington, DC: Office of the Inspector General, Region X.

Wright, J., & Weber, E. (1987). *Homelessness and health.* New York: McGraw-Hill.

Yates, G., MacKenzie, R., Pennbridge, J., & Cohen, E. (1988). A risk profile comparison of runaway and non-runaway youth. *American Journal of Public Health, 78,* 820–821.

Assessment and Treatment of Homeless Mentally Ill Adults

16

Paul Koegel, Daniel Sherman

CHAPTER HIGHLIGHTS

- As many as one third of our nation's homeless adults suffer from severe mental illness. The mentally ill homeless have multiple problems including basic survival needs that may take priority over their mental health concerns.
- Treating the mentally ill homeless requires a sensitivity to the concerns and values of a distinctive subgroup of the mentally ill as well as a broadly defined concept of treatment.
- Limited resources often compel mental health programs for the homeless to triage clients, serving only those with major mental illnesses such as schizophrenia, major depression, or bipolar disorder.
- Homelessness itself can lead to behaviors that are symptomatic of mental illness, making diagnosis difficult. Alcohol and drug abuse further complicate the task of diagnosis of mental illness among the homeless.
- Assessment of the mentally ill homeless includes a short screening interview, followed by a more lengthy detailed intake to ascertain the client's psychosocial history, substance abuse and psychiatric symptoms, current needs, and social functioning and skills.
- To treat the homeless mentally ill effectively a continuum of innovative services is required that should include outreach,

drop-in centers, mental health clinics, and a variety of housing options.

- Case management of services for the homeless mentally ill should be directed at both stabilizing their symptoms and their lives.
- Mental health clinics for the homeless should be accessible in terms of location, hours, and scheduling; include a range of psychiatric and outreach personnel who work in "treatment teams"; and should ensure security for clinic personnel.

INTRODUCTION

As many as one third of our nation's homeless adults suffer from a variety of severe mental illness disorders including schizophrenia and major affective disorder (Arce & Vergare, 1984; Robertson, in press; Tessler & Dennis, 1989). Although the process of de-institutionalization is most often cited as the explanation for the many mentally ill homeless (Lamb, 1984), the primary cause has more to do with broader economic changes that have left an increasing number of poor people—among whom the mentally ill are most vulnerable—competing for a shrinking number of low-income housing units (Hopper & Hamburg, 1986). The result is that a particularly needy group of people experience the full gamut of problems that afflict all homeless people, but have much more trouble meeting their needs because of their psychiatric illness (Bassuk, 1984; Tessler & Dennis, 1989; Segal, Baumohl, & Johnson, 1977).

In many important ways, homeless mentally ill individuals are similar to their non–mentally ill homeless counterparts. They tend to be young, nonwhite males. They are largely long-term residents of the communities in which they are found. They overwhelmingly cite economic factors and family conflict as the primary reasons for their homelessness. They also tend to have problems with alcohol and drugs in very high numbers. They also have more entrenched histories of homelessness, a higher degree of mobility, more strained relationships with family members, and more difficulties in maintaining employment. As a group, they are neither receiving the disability support to which they are entitled nor the mental health services they need. In addition, they are arrested far more often than their non–mentally ill counterparts and spend more time in jail. By default, it seems, the criminal justice system is becoming responsible for their care (Morrissey & Dennis, 1986; Tessler & Dennis, 1989).

Increasingly, it is realized that the population of homeless mentally ill individuals is not comprised only of "stereotypic" individuals (i.e. isolated, disheveled, psychotic street dwellers). Rather, the mentally ill homeless also consist of much higher-functioning individuals (whom are virtually indistinguishable from their non–mentally ill brethren), as well as myraid others who fall somewhere in between these two extremes. Moreover, it has become clear that the proportion of homeless mentally ill persons who reject all services is very small, and that the failure of this population to obtain needed services is most often the result of structural, procedural and psychological barriers to care (Koegel, in press; Plapinger, 1988).

We propose that mental health services to the homeless mentally ill must rest on a broader base of knowledge than is traditionally required of the mental health professional. Although mental health diagnostic criteria and traditional treatment strategies are fundamental, the practitioner needs "hands-on" experience with mental illness in the homeless setting to help this population successfully. A sensitivity to the concerns and values of this distinctive subgroup of the mentally ill and a willingness to entertain a broader conception of treatment are also essential.

ASSESSMENT

Mental health programs for the homeless, owing to limited resources, are usually forced to triage clients, accepting for ongoing treatment only those individuals with major mental illnesses of schizophrenia, major depression, or bipolar disorder. Screening is therefore critical, not only because it helps identify a person's problem and course of treatment, but also because it determines who is eligible for services. Individuals with problems such as personality disorders or personal crises are referred to other, frequently minimal, community resources. This is regrettable, because many people with personality and anxiety disorders could profit from professional mental health services. These patients usually require psychotherapy as well as possible medications, however, and treatment is usually of longer duration, frequently with a need for psychodynamic "uncovering." Given the cost-intensive nature of this work, these patient's ultimately go unserved.

Crisis therapy will be involved in addressing an individual's presenting complaint. Although this may entail simple instrumental case management (i.e., establishing an appointment with a welfare worker), in all likelihood, the intervention will also focus on the individual's perception of his or her own abilities and level of need. Focusing on the individual's adaptive ego strength and discussing alternative coping strategies should be considered as an integral, ethical process in any referral to outside services when interviewing with higher-functioning or axis II (per DSM-3) individuals. Additionally, a factual explanation regarding the severity of symptoms required to meet criteria for services cannot only aid less disturbed individuals to feel more accepting of their situation but may lead them to identify and refer more severely mentally ill who meet criteria to the clinic for services.

The coexistence of homelessness and mental illness poses enormous diagnostic challenges to providers. For example, the skills that homeless individuals have developed to adapt to their very difficult circumstances may occasionally be mistaken as evidence of mental illness. Fear of being followed may seem like bizarre or paranoid behavior to a clinician. It may be a sensible and hard-learned adjustment to life on the streets, however, where muggers gravitate monthly to check-cashing stores in search of those with disability entitlements. In addition, many homeless individuals are often suffering from severe substance abuse problems that can mask, or masquerade as, psychiatric disorder. For example, crack cocaine users have frequently been misdiagnosed as both paranoid and manic.

Conditions of homelessness may actually lead to behaviors that are symptomatic of mental illness, making it difficult to determine whether observed symptoms are caused by mental illness or present circumstances (Koegel & Burnam, in press). The prolonged stress and constant assaults to self-esteem that homeless individuals endure, for instance, over time may produce transient disorientation, personality disorganization, or even paranoid psychoses. In a similar manner, residual symptoms of schizophrenia may be exacerbated by daily life stress.

CASE STUDY

A 30-year-old woman was so disoriented when first observed at a mental health clinic that she was involuntarily hospitalized on a 72-hour hold. A month-long stay in a crisis treatment facility, however, found her completely stabilized without medication. The woman was diagnosed as having a reactive psychosis brought on by the trauma of homelessness and, with help, she eventually was able to move into her own apartment and find a job.

The overwhelming array of basic needs experienced by the homeless adult further complicates the assessment process. Many clients presenting complaints do not include a report of symptomatology nor need for medication. Rather, the primary request is a need for housing, food, clothing, or help in securing public income entitlements. Such individuals may feel that *these* are their most serious problems, not the voices they hear or the strange beliefs they hold. The clinician must start by responding to the client's immediate need, as well as continuously observing and listening for key psychopathological symptoms.

In our experience, assessment works best if broken into two stages: screening and detailed intake.

Screening

During the screening interview, which may last for no more than 20–30 minutes), the goal is to determine whether the prospective client is suffering from symptoms of severe mental illness such as severe depression, psychoses, or suicide intent. Usually, the screening process will include determining the clients' presenting problem, medical problems, income sources, where they live, past and current medications, past and current substance abuse history, past psychiatric history, and a determination of their current mental status.

It should be noted that, although desirable, the screening process does not have to be complete. An individual who stumbles into a clinic with alcohol on his or her breath, requesting a bus ticket, need not answer all the screening questions to be told to return sober. Likewise, an older individual who, in a rational manner, denies a psychiatric history and requests medical aid, need not be queried regarding mental status or arrest history.

Even if individuals present in the preceding manner, a clinician may, because of the client's appearance, still wish to evaluate mental status, however. Behavior observation must frequently provide the clinician with a sense of the homeless person's existent mental condition. A demented individual's inability to dress properly or move facilely, a suicidal individual's tears, or the sweating palms or labored breathing of an individual with an anxiety disorder may all lead the clinician to probe beyond the presenting problem. Attention to behavior details is vital.

A homeless individual may wear multiple layers of clothing for warmth in the winter; however, usually only a psychotic individual will do this in the summer months (often with a mismatched color scheme). Although the possibility remains that women dressed in this manner are engaged in a strategy to protect themselves against sexual assault (Koegel, 1987).

The screening should proceed from the least intrusive to more personal questions. For example, clinicians might first ask whether the patient receives financial aid Veteran's benefits, or is on Medicare or Medicaid. Once ascertaining that benefits remain intact, then the clinician can seek to determine the specific disability. Eventually, a time line regarding the areas of psychiatric disturbance, substance abuse, and arrest history should be obtained. This time line is vital. For example, among individuals with schizophrenia, substance use and arrests usually follow, rather than precede, the first schizophrenic break. Similarly, if an individual reports a first episode of major depression that preceded his use of substances, the likelihood is greater that the patient has been self-medicating and that the problem is not solely substance related. Likewise, if an individual first heard voices long before she was ever homeless, her symptoms are probably psychiatrically relevant even if they might be hypothesized as environmentally "stress related."

In this vein, it is important to never take the phrase "I hear voices" at face value. Observations of a client's reaction to active auditory hallucinations (difficult to replicate consistently when not psychotic) are vital. Does the patient really hear a "voice" and not a "thought"? Does it only happen under severe stress or at all hours of the day? When does the individual hear voices? Is it only when alone at night, or only when she is in a particular hotel room known for its drug activity? Likewise, the phrase "people are out to get me" should always be explored further, because a moderate dose of paranoia is often healthy in the environments in which homeless individuals live.

If the screening process rules out major mental illness, clinic mental health services must usually be denied. Understandably, clients who are refused services will at times express a great deal of anger that is neither easily deflected nor ignored. Information should always be provided as to basic goal setting as well as where individuals might go to meet their subsistence and other basic needs, (showers, job centers, welfare offices). This also tends to decrease, or at least channel, the patient's frustration. Whenever appropriate, referrals should be made to a low-fee or free counsling clinic that provides therapy services to those without a disabling major mental illness.

Detailed Intake

A more lengthy *intake* of approximately 60 to 90 minutes should follow the initial screening to flesh out further the client's psychosocial history, past and current substance abuse, psychiatric symptoms, current needs, and current social functioning and skills. Such information can then be used to refine the client's diagnosis and to create a treatment plan. In a sense, the intake is simply a more detailed version of the screening.

After discussing the client's presenting complaint, the interview should then assess the individual's current living conditions. These issues are important for several reasons. First, they provide an additional chance to discuss issues that are meaningful to the client (in almost all cases, the client has concerns about his or her environment). More important, it opens up opportunities to respond to the client's immediate concerns with instrumental aid and, thereby, cement rapport and pave the way for a more successful interaction.

The clinician should always listen to assess the client's presenting complaints. Be attentive if the client needs medical treatment, has a need for new eye glasses, and so on. Determine whether a bus pass might make the person's life somewhat easier, and be responsive to complaints regarding public entitlements. These concerns demonstrate to clients that you are working for them. It also allows you to determine how logical and goal directed or manipulative the client may be. The client's level of judgment and insight can be quickly assessed if, when without shelter or food, their consuming concern is to obtain the telephone number of the president. By giving the client access to the telephone to attempt to call the White House, however, you may increase their trust in you and in your attempt to address their needs.

Meeting basic needs of homeless mentally ill individuals must be seen as the first step in successful mental health interventions. Programs for the homeless mentally ill in New York City found that the single best predictor of a successful mental health referral was a successful housing placement (Barrow, 1988).

The client's living conditions also reveal something about the client's current adaptation and level of functioning. Finally, it also reveals cues as to whether environment plays a role in what the individual's current experiences are. For instance, a report of vegetative symptoms of depression (sleep or appetite disturbance) may be attributed to the difficult conditions that exist in some mission facilities.

Once a foundation of trust has been established, it is then easier to ask a client about his or her mental health symptoms. In most ways, conducting a mental status examination is no different with the homeless population though, as indicated earlier. It is critical to attend to both content and *context* in evaluating what you hear. This is particularly true when trying to assess the presence of a major depressive episode. It is vital to observe the client's behavior when assessing for major depression. How does the client relate to you? Does he laugh at a joke, make good eye contact over time, or demonstrate normal rate of speech? Or, despite every attempt, does he remain downcast, dejected, with slowed motor movements, minimal speech, or wringing of hands? Does he maintain pride on his appearance, or has his decreased self-esteem led to observable decreased hygiene that frequently parallels the presence of vegetative symptoms of depression?

Similarly, it is vital to realize that many symptoms of depression (e.g., sleep disturbance, weight loss, social isolation) may be affected by homelessness. Homeless individuals should be asked when they last enjoyed successive nights of comfortable (nonmission) sleep and had access to regular meals. A historical assessment of vegetative symptoms should include questions regarding this period before a final diagnosis is made. Knowing that a client has slept in the street for the last month may place his complaints of sleep disturbance in a different light, especially if he was sleeping well immediately before this when lodging was provided by his parents. Knowing that he has been scavenging in the garbage for food may lead you to interpret his weight loss differently. Realizing that perhaps "mission life" has led the patient to lose the cues that allow him to know what day it is may help you understand an apparent disorientation to time, while retaining the ability to make daily appointments with you.

It is also essential to determine whether a substance use disorder was present before, coexists with, or is the result of psychiatric symptoms. In most instances, questions will be received more equitably than one might imagine, especially if they are asked in a nonjudgmental way. Clinicians should remember that many clients use substances to self-medicate feelings of low self-esteem, anxiety, depression, and even hallucinations. This awareness should be specifically conveyed to clients before clinicians take a substance use history.

Substance use can seriously complicate the task of diagnosis, especially regarding major affective disorders. A client may present with symptoms of paranoia or mania that are actually caused by the crack cocaine he smoked before entering the clinic. When drug use is suspected (for example, when manic behavior is accompanied by dilated or constricted pupils, sweating, and a flushed appearance), ask if such symptoms are present when the individual is *not* using drugs. If a client appears high, recommend that it would be best to return on a day when the client is "clean." Alternatively, it may be possible to delay seeing an individual for several hours until they come down. Under such circumstances, it is possible to feel more assured that observed behavior is not directly tied to drug use.

Mental health diagnosis is even more complicated when drinking is involved, in the context of alcohol abuse. A clinician should explain it would first be better for the client to first enter a detoxification program for 30 days to see if that improves his mood. This may be unreasonable, because both the mental health and substance abuse systems tend not to take responsibility for dually diagnosed clients. Whenever possible, it is best to refer such individuals to programs for persons with dual diagnoses of substance abuse and major mental illness. Unfortunately, such programs are rare and have long waiting lists. In the absence of such programs, the clinician is faced with the choice of either trying to work with the client despite the diagnostic uncertainty caused by the alcoholism, or helping him enter and stay in a detoxification program. This might mean consulting with alcohol program staff and maintaining contact with the client. In the absence of this additional support, the chances of the individual falling between the cracks of the two systems are high.

A detailed history is the cornerstone for establishing an accurate diagnosis. As noted earlier, a time line regarding the appearance of psychiatric symptoms is crucial. A complete history addresses the client's educational background including job history, longest job, last job, and reasons for that job ending. This yields a sense of the person's potential, provides information for Supplemental Security Income evaluations, and reveals cues that may help distinguish someone with a personality disorder from someone with a major mental illness. A residential history can provide insight into living arrangements that have worked in the past, and possibly will again in the future. The social history should assess social relationships during the school years with peers and teachers (helpful in diagnosing antisocial personalities), as well as assessing family relationships, friends, and marriages. All the preceding information can provide clues about the person's initial illness, severity of symptoms, as well as may suggest potential support for the client or collateral sources of information in the clinician.

CASE STUDY

A homeless man presented at the Skid Row Mental Health Services complaining of angry voices. Further questioning determined that the "voices" sounded like one person, a past family member, and was limited to either only calling his name or, on occasion, saying, "You are no good!" (mirroring the patient's low self-esteem). These voices occurred only at specific times (when he was alone, and thinking at night about his life) and lasted for brief intervals of 5 seconds. An in-depth social history revealed that he had the social skills to remain married, although he was plagued by frequent but brief anger outbursts. He had a long history of anger reactions from age 13, leading to placement with juvenile authorities. According to his wife, the voices began after multiple LSD use at age 19, and he had used cocaine during their marriage. His diagnosis was one of a mixed personality disorder with atypical psychosis, hypothesized to result from substance use. He was encouraged to seek therapy as well as involvement in Cocaine Anonymous to increase social supports.

Finally, a history should include a list of medications that the individual has taken for mental health reasons. These provide important diagnostic clues. In addition, it may be possible to ask the client which medications have worked most effectively for him in the past. Often, clients know that they have responded better to a particular medication at a particular dosage, or that they have experienced side effects from another. Enlisting their perspective and knowledge is another effective way of bolstering rapport and obtaining needed information for diagnosis and treatment. If a client insists only on valium, a personality disorder must be considered.

In general, as with the screening process, intake questions should proceed from the least intrusive to the more personal. At times, it may be necessary to display a great deal of patience in awaiting answers, especially from clients who are fearful or withdrawn. Whenever possible, it helps to use the vernacular. It is also critical to work efficiently, because a client's tolerance of formal interviews may be limited. Mental health examinations and histories can be structured so that one leapfrogs from one area to another based on the client's response to a question. Efficiency, however, should never be pursued at the expense of listening to what the client has to say. Some amount of time must be allocated to allow clients to pursue their own agendas, no matter how tangential they may seem. Being listened to is not an experience that these individuals consistently enjoy in their day-to-day lives, and is the simplest way to build rapport and obtain diagnostic information.

In addition to client verbal responses, the client's behavior helps the clinician assess mental status and functioning. Concentration and memory tasks are unnecessary in a client who is on time for a formal intake appointment that was scheduled a week ago, maintains good eye contact, and informs you that he must be back at the mission by 2:00 p.m. to obtain a bed ticket. The clinician may ask other pertinent questions (such as addresses or telephone numbers of past work supervisors) to document for Supplemental Security Income benefits. Clients who are too disoriented, withdrawn, or unable to communicate effectively may have difficulty engaging in a long intake procedure. Even when a client is able to communicate effectively, behavioral observation can provide information that corrects client self-report. In clinics with a central waiting area, the clinician can often gain significant information by observing, unobtrusively, clients in the waiting room.

CASE STUDY

A homeless woman's strange behavior was representative of a "classic" psychosis and quickly led to a diagnosis and treatment plan. Dressed in multilayer clothing and wearing layers of cosmetics, she entered the clinic, loudly demanding that the clinic radio be disconnected to end her perceived harassment by the American Medical Association. She reported that this harassment tended to decrease when she took Haldol and screamed that she would accept a prescription for this medication from any "qualified technician" to stop the voices that "queer her." Her statements were sprinkled with obscenities, and her associations were loose. The clinician quickly isolated her in a private room and wrote a formal description of her mental status without asking the patient any questions. This allowed for medication to be prescribed quickly by injection. Intake details were added 5 days later, after she had stabilized on medication.

In addition to observation, the complete evaluation should solicit the perspective of others who know the client or have known the client in the past. Family members, other mental health agencies, detoxification programs, and welfare workers may all be valuable sources of insight into the client, as can state and county computerized management information systems. Such information is especially valuable when clients are unable or unwilling to offer details about their histories.

Finally, laboratory work may also provide definitive answers to certain questions. Urine and blood tests should be used if the patient is taking lithium levels or to assess the presence of illicit drugs (with the client's permission). In rare cases, HIV testing may be indicated to confirm a suspected diagnosis of AIDS-related dementia. Ideally, clinics should have the capacity to draw and analyze blood on site. Clients will seldom return to the clinic if the laboratory technician is not currently present, nor will they usually go to another hospital or clinic for a blood test.

In general, the assessment of homeless mentally ill clients must be sufficiently comprehensive to screen eligible individuals, rule out environmental factors, and establish the relationship between highly comorbid syndromes. At the same time, clinicians should recognize and respond to the self-perceived needs of homeless persons, both as a way of establishing rapport and as a first step in the provision of effective treatment.

TREATMENT

It is impossible to discuss treating homeless mentally ill adults without emphasizing several points: Homeless mentally ill adults have strong opinions regarding what they want and how it should be provided; they have *multiple* needs that must be met concurrently; and they have learned from years of past experience to be leery of the mental health profession. Given these realities, an unprecedented level of patience may be required before positive results can be obtained.

Given the heterogeneity of the homeless mentally ill population and the multiplicity of their needs, traditional community mental health treatment by itself will simply not be effective. We now know that a *continuum* of services is required. This includes outreach to those who are isolated or simply too floridly psychotic to access services at all; drop-in centers that meet instrumental and social needs on as-needed basis and provide a foundation for more formal mental health treatment; and clinics capable of providing rapid access to medication, group therapy, and related services. A continuum of housing options is also needed, including support for those who find it difficult to leave the streets immediately, congregate living quarters that provide minimal restrictions or demands, transitional living programs geared toward moving clients toward independent living, low-income rooms or apartments in locales that allow for social integration and a sense of community, and skilled nursing facilities or hospitals for the markedly impaired and consistently gravely disabled.

Outreach

A traditional clinic usually waits for clients to present themselves. Many homeless mentally ill adults, however, are too dysfunctional, alienated, or afraid to enter a clinic unassisted. These individuals, if they are to receive services at all, must be served where they are found.

For safety as well as for logistical reasons, outreach should be conducted in pairs. Outreach workers can engage homeless individuals by offering cigarettes, small food items, blankets, clothing, and any other items that a homeless individual may prize. These are offered as a means of establishing a relationship. The approach to a prospective client should be quiet, respectful, and completely unpressured, maintaining a nonthreatening distance. Because some clients may be unpredictably violent, outreach workers should ensure that they and the prospective client always have an exit pathway if intimidated. Outreach workers should be trained in the management of assaultive behavior as well.

Workers should identify themselves as the "outreach team" rather than the "mental health outreach team," because many individuals will be especially suspicious of those attached to the mental health system. Offers of assistance should be couched in general terms, such as "Is there anything you want? Is there anything you need, like food, shelter, or medication?" A relationship is best initiated by responding to what the client wants and allowing the initiation of mental health treatment to await the development of trust.

Patience must be a byword and progress measured in exceptionally small units. It may take weeks of contact to just get a person to establish eye contact. Getting them to accept a blanket or food may be weeks away; entering a car for a health clinic appointment may take months; accepting mental health services may take even longer. Here, more than at any point in the treatment continuum, intervention must proceed at the pace set by the client whenever possible. Only then can a viable relationship emerge. With enough time, it may be possible to guide the individual into an indoor shelter arrangement or drop-in center, and into a clinic where more formal mental health services can be provided.

Given the skittishness, fear, and distrust of many clients, as well as their abhorrence of institutions, hospitalization should be avoided unless absolutely necessary. If hospitalization is deemed necessary, one option is to have the police or a psychiatric emergency team manage the task so that the outreach worker's relationship with the client is not jeopardized. If the outreach worker handles the hospitalization, he or she should accompany the client in the ambulance and continue to visit the client in the hospital. This gives the outreach worker a chance to interact with a medicated, and stabilized, client, as well as demonstrate her commitment to the clients. Also, if someone is interested in the client, the hospital may provide better treatment and be more willing to involve the outreach worker in discharge planning.

Outreach also includes consultation services to other community agencies who serve the homeless. Outreach workers may often run groups in shelters, soup kitchens, or day-centers. They can provide staff trainings on recognizing and managing symptoms of mental illness or even conduct on-site assessments of clients about whom staff members are concerned. Staff from outside facilities learn, through this contact, to refer appropriate clients to the clinic (see chapter 4 by Smith on outreach clinics.)

In most mental health clinics (which tend to be filled to capacity shortly after opening their doors), a tension will always exist between the importance of reaching out to needy individuals and the recognition that the clinic is frequently unable to serve adequately even those who come to the clinic themselves. When outreach occurs, it is critical to ensure that outreach clients be given priority so that their act of courage does not go unrewarded. Marking charts with a special priority label or color is one way of ensuring that this will occur.

CASE STUDY

A homeless man had been observed by outreach workers standing at one particular parking lot for 2 weeks. Contact with this man was initially nonverbal, consisting of nonverbal refusals of food; however, he did accept a blanket. A parking attendant reported that the man had refused food for the past 2 months, although occasionally ate from trash cans. His hygiene was poor; in addition, his motor behavior and speed were slow, typical of the apathy and lack of self-worth found in many major depressive disorders. He finally spoke to outreach workers and eventually agreed to ride with them to the clinic. He refused to leave the car, but a clinic worker walked out of the clinic to meet him. Subsequent outreach contacts with this clinic worker were arranged. After three more automobile trips, Danny was finally convinced to accept housing and, eventually, medicine to help with his "memory problems." Six months after formal treatment, he was reunited with his family who he had last contacted 11 years earlier.

Drop-In Centers

Drop-in centers represent the next step on the treatment continuum. Ideally, a drop-in center is housed in a storefront facility that is centrally located. The center should be a low-demand place where individuals can wander in and out easily, and should provide the non-mental health–related services prized by homeless individuals. These are, in and of themselves, legitimate mental health services and can facilitate more formal mental health treatment. Meals, clothing, and daytime beds are an excellent attraction, as are services such as providing a mailing address, offering assistance in obtaining financial entitlements, allowing clients to deposit and draw money from their checks, providing linkages to other services, and providing daily living skills training. Above all else, drop-in centers should provide a comfortable environment in which people can get off the streets, sit quietly, or socialize with others.

Ultimately, a drop-in center will be most effective if it is either attached to, or has close relations with, a mental health clinic. Under such circumstances, drop-in center staff can capitalize on the trust and rapport that they build over time with clients to introduce to them the possibility of therapy or medication. Likewise, the clinic can direct clients to the drop-in center. When referrals are made, the service provider should accompany the client to the new facility to ease the client's anxiety and introduce the client to people there.

Clinics

Clinics that serve homeless mentally ill adults primarily conduct structured assessments and provide mental health treatment. As medication is usually central to the treatment of chronic mental disorders, clinics should ideally have a pharmacy either on site or nearby. Additionally, a double-locked storage facility for medications is important to monitor medication compliance and provide safe storage for pills that may be lost, stolen, or lose efficacy. Clinics should also have the capacity to provide intramuscular injections of medication for those who have trouble maintaining a treatment regimen, as well as liquid medication for acute manifestations of symptoms.

Many homeless mentally ill individuals are extremely reluctant to take medication. They may feel that the side effects are distasteful and stigmatizing, or that medication interferes with their ability to react quickly to threatening street situations. In some cases, a client's refusal of medication stems from a feeling that being dependent on medication compromises integrity, defines them as impaired, and results in behavior governed by something external. In still other cases, it is because delusions can be adaptive

Even though the decision to refuse medication may be rational from the client's viewpoint, the clinician may still believe that the client's survival of life concerns are best served by medication. The attractiveness of medication may be increased if certain resources are made contingent on the client's willingness to maintain a medication regimen. This is not to say that a client's access to subsistence and other services should be tied to his or her willingness to accept medication. Certain resources, such as a transitional housing program that provides independent work, may in reality not be appropriate unless the client is sufficiently stabilized, however. The lure of the service can be used as an inducement to convince the client to take prescribed drugs.

Mental health services must involve more than the disbursement of medication. Therapy, though not the kind of insight therapy that is usually associated with mental health professionals, should also be offered. Clinics should attempt to provide both individual and group therapy. More disturbed patients may, in fact, require individual work to prepare them for group work. Therapy requires the counselor to meet regularly with the client to help set goals, support their attempts to meet these goals, and monitor their progress. Goals must be adjusted to the functioning level of the client, and in some cases will involve nothing more than showing up for a Supplemental Security Income hearing or a transitional housing program interview, or maintaining a specified lithium level. Therapy consists of taking small steps and reinforcing them. For higher-functioning clients, more expansive and interpersonal group therapy might be indicated. Above all, mental health clinics should recognize that services such as money management, socialization, housing, entitlements, and health care are legitimate mental health services that must be provided, either directly, or in conjunction with affiliated providers and clinics.

Housing

Mental health treatment will not fare very well unless a concomitant effort is made to stabilize clients and reduce the stress in their lives. Thus, low-cost, decent housing represents a critical component of mental health services. Sadly, the lack of safe, affordable housing is one of the biggest frustrations a service provider will face (Plapinger, 1988).

A continuum of housing options for the homeless mentally ill is needed. Although some individuals may immediately accept any number of housing options, others may have spent so much time living on the streets that the thought of being indoors is frightening and strange. These clients may not be ready to move inside and may require, instead, help in making their lives on the streets more comfortable. Eventually, they may be willing to move into housing that is extremely low demand and that allows easy access to the outdoors, even in the middle of the night. Later, they may enter transitional living programs that include skill building, serviced housing in the community, or low-cost, independent housing.

Just as there are rational elements to the decision not to take medication, there are often very compelling reasons for people's housing choices, even those that do not, at first glance, make sense. Some homeless adults reject a stable board-and-care facility in favor of a more uncertain life on the streets because the boring, highly structured life-style associated with institutional settings is antithetical to the high value they place on autonomy and self-determination. Some homeless adults choose not to purchase housing in available SRO hotels because they realize how unsafe and unsanitary such rooms may be, or because they want to spend their money on other things (such as cigarettes, movie tickets, other personal goods). They may also fear that living in an SRO will leave them isolated and invisible. Finally, the homeless adult may have established social ties and a relationship with a community on the streets that keeps him or her from accepting an exemplary housing placement on the other side of town. Thus, housing options must not only be diverse, but also attuned to client concerns, inner resources, and course of treatment. As is true with services in general, where a housing choice bears a hidden but unacceptable price, it will either be rejected or short-lived.

CASE MANAGEMENT AND CONTINUITY OF CARE

Case Management

The case manager is the glue holding the disparate elements of treatment together and molding them into one coherent plan. Case management assigns responsibility for coordinating needed services to one person. The case manager advocates on the client's behalf and steers, and even physically accompanies, the client through the maze of subsistence, mental health, substance abuse, public entitlement and health services. In a sense, the case manager is a broker between the client and the system at large, helping to articulate and meet needs, ensuring continuity of care, and participating in ongoing problem solving.

The particularities of case management have been reviewed extensively elsewhere (Rog, Andranovich, & Rosenblum, 1987; see also chapter 3 by Cousineau, Casanova, & Erlenbusch) and will not be repeated here. It is important to stress, however, that case management, if done effectively, is a very arduous and complicated task; 12 clients are probably an ideal case load. Unfortunately, limited resources may prevent this ideal from being reached. A strong argument can be made that it is better to have fewer cases managed well than many cases managed poorly. Establishing two separate case management "tracks" with one being for intensive case management may be the best compromise many overwhelmed clinics can make.

Continuity

Once an individual is brought into a system of care, every effort should be made to assure that such care continues. As a group, the homeless mentally ill are not generally rooted to one place by residential ties, are often skittish and easily scared away, and can easily get lost between the cracks of the social service network. As a result, continuity of care is often lost.

As indicated earlier, the case manager position is perhaps the best guarantee of continuity. Continuity, however, can be ensured on a structural level as well, especially when new systems of care are being designed to meet the needs of homeless mentally ill adults. Ideally, outreach teams, clinics, drop-in centers, shelters, crisis centers, transitional living centers, serviced SRO hotels, and scatter-site housing are all integrated into one system, either because they are united under a single administrative umbrella or because key players have established guidelines for working in tandem. When this is the case, clinicians and service providers have the resources to respond to clients' needs immediately, and to advance them along the continuum of housing and treatment. When this is not the case, the case manager and clinic staff have a greater responsibility to forge strong referral ties and ongoing relationships with other agencies or facilities to piece together an integrated system of care.

Within an agency, continuity of care can be advanced by ensuring that every staff member has a vested interest in treatment at every step along the range of offered services. This can be accomplished by rotating people across tasks so that every staff member experiences every segment of treatment at one time or another. In a clinic, for instance, a social worker may do outreach on some days, assessment on other days, housing placement on yet other days, and case management throughout. Such a staff member will not only have a better sense of the difficulty of each stage of treatment, but may be more committed to serving particular clients by virtue of having had past experience with them at a different point in time.

Continuity of care goes beyond the issue of what happens while the individual is being served in the present; it must address the issue of how past treatment leads into what will happen in the future. This area is perhaps more problematic than any. Finding service providers who have treated the client in the past can be time-consuming, and thus often impractical, but is inevitably rewarding in its informational yield and development of further treatment plans. Ensuring future continuity is easier, at least on a local level. When a person is referred to a new local system of care, such as a psychosocial rehabilitation agency that has its own case managers, the previous case manager can remain in contact until the client is completely settled in the new system, brokering any problems between client and new case worker, and providing cotherapy with the new case worker to support the client during a stressful transitional period. If an individual suddenly decides to relocate, the task is more difficult. The clinician or case manager can at least telephone ahead to the client's intended destination to locate agencies that can serve him or her in the new setting. Ideally, an actual transfer of responsibility should be negotiated so that someone is waiting for that individual when he or she steps off the bus, though this is only rarely feasible.

CLINIC LOGISTICS

Although the kind of treatment that homeless mentally ill individuals require spans many settings, generally the traditional aspects of treatment will occur in some kind of clinic setting. Operating a mental health clinic for homeless mentally ill adults carries with it its own set of logistical challenges.

Physical Layout

Storefronts, as a rule, are far more accessible and far less threatening than imposing settings that require an individual to negotiate hallways, stairs, or elevators. Similarly, an internal layout that consists of work stations that protect the privacy of dyadic interactions, but are also open to the view of others will be far less threatening to both clients and staff. Small, isolated rooms with closed doors are ill suited to this population: Clients may feel trapped by the claustrophobic feel of such offices, whereas staff may feel isolated from potential sources of support should they be necessary.

Hours

Most clinics find mornings to be the busiest time. An ideal time to open is around 7:00 a.m., by which time missions and shelters have closed their doors, and people are starting their days. Unlike drop-in centers, which would ideally be open 7 days a week, a clinic need not necessarily remain open beyond 4:00 p.m. Some thought might even be given to rotating staff across 4 10-hour days. This way, staff would have 3 consecutive days off per week, and be less likely to experience burnout.

Off-hours psychiatric emergencies can be handled by local psychiatric emergency teams or the police. Alternatively, though more expensive, emergencies can be addressed by a rotating around-the-clock mobile emergency team that can admit people to a small crisis shelter, if available, or transport them to the local psychiatric emergency department. Case management crises can be handled either by a telephone answering machine informing clients when staff will return and where they can turn for help in the interim, or an on-call system in which one or two case managers cover all clients on a rotating basis.

Scheduling

Ideally, the capacity for both scheduled appointments and walk-ins should be available. Appointments are often difficult for homeless mentally ill people to manage, either because of their illness or because of the exigencies of the homeless life-style. Many clients are completely capable of keeping appointments, however, and should be expected to do so as this adds to making clinic functioning more predictable. When clients are kept waiting, the clinic should do all it can to make them comfortable and to acknowledge that they are being inconvenienced.

Team Composition

Team composition will vary depending on a clinic's size, goals, and resources. Because people have such diverse needs, many disciplines should be represented on the treatment team. At a minimum, a psychiatrist will be needed to prescribe medication; a psychologist to aid with diagnosis, testing, and Supplemental Security Income evaluations; a psychiatric nurse for insight into medical problems; and community workers who are out on the streets maintaining contact with the target population. Administrative and secretarial support staff will be required as well. Clinics should expect, however, that responsibilities will overlap and that everyone will be doing a little of everything. For example, a clinical social worker can aid psychiatrists in providing mental status reports for Supplemental Security Income evaluations; a psychologist can engage in outreach.

Coordinating Team Efforts

Frequent meetings between team members are absolutely essential to ensure that efforts are coordinated. Case presentations in which diagnosis, treatment plan, and progress are laid out should occur regularly, as should briefer updates on what is going on with

particular clients. Once clients actually enter the clinic, good charting is an extremely important way of ensuring that staff is presenting
a consistent front. Charts should contain progress notes and a section
in which staff can jot down decisions relating to the client. If a client
stops by while a case worker is on outreach and reports, for instance,
that the case worker said he could withdraw more than his weekly
allowance, another staff member should be able to look at a chart or
some other common information-sharing place (e.g., a blackboard)
and confirm that this is true.

Staff Turnover

Because of the overwhelming stress of working with such a needy
population, staff is at high risk for burnout. To keep staff turnover at
a minimum, administrators must create an environment that nur-
tures and supports those who work within it. Staff meetings are a
must. Process meetings could also be instituted to enhance opportunities for staff to share feelings, frustrations, and potential strategies for handling problems with one another. Regular retreats in
which issues regarding working with the homeless population are
thrashed out can be effective as well as the simpler, but so often
neglected, strategy of communicating to staff how valuable their
work is and how much they are appreciated. Scheduling opportunities for seminars also adds to the staffs' investment in their positions.

Security

The issue of whether uniformed, armed security guards should be
present in a clinic is a controversial one. Proponents of armed guards
argue that security is necessary to make staff feel safe. Opponents
argue that when symbols of violence are present, the likelihood of
aggression is increased, and that security guards do not always have
the training to be effective in a mental health setting. The sense of
security engendered by guards is a false one, opponents claim.

When the decision is made to retain a security guard, the person
must be one who remains on-site consistently and must answer to
clinic staff, not to an outside security firm. Special training should be
required to include empathy training, limit setting, ways to talk
people down, the application of holds, and placement of restraints on
people. It should be made clear that the role of the security person is
to help contain clients who are having difficulty containing them-

selves. At all times, it should be clear to a security guard that if the clinician instructs the guard to back off, he or she will do so. At the same time, the clinician must feel confident that, if a client becomes assaultive, the security guard will intervene.

CONCLUSION

The profoundly disturbing recognition that thousands of chronically mentally ill individuals now live on the streets has led many to call for a return to institutionalization—that is, to involuntarily restrict those who appear unable to care for themselves to settings in which others can care for them. Deinstitutionalization, we are told, is a social experiment that failed and a social policy that must be reversed, not only for the sake of the persons whose lives it has affected but for the communities that are confronted daily by their unsightly presence.

It seems to us, as it does to many others, that deinstitutionalization is better viewed as an experiment that has yet to be tested properly, making any conclusions as to its relative worth quite premature. By neither supporting community mental health at the level it requires nor attending to the issue of where the poorer members of our society will live, we have spent years fostering conditions that have condemned many chronically mentally ill individuals to the most marginal of existences. It strikes us as unfair to blame them for the circumstances in which they find themselves and to rectify our errors by forcing on them a set of conditions they abhor.

A more logical approach, we think, is to give deinstitutionalization the chance it never had by providing services that are consistent with the skills, values, and beliefs of homeless mentally ill clients, recognizing all the while that attitudes that took years to create might take years to be remediated. This approach is, primarily, based on a belief in respecting the inherent dignity of individuals, especially those who have an illness that they did not chose and that society chose first to warehouse and then ignore. After a protracted period of patiently offering homeless mentally ill individuals quality care, we may be better able to assess whether they are capable of choosing wisely for themselves. Until then, our responsibility is to serve them as best we can, improving our services as we learn more about who they are, what they want, and what they need. Finally, we need to *prevent* further occurrences of homelessness among this vulnerable population as we better understand how this social tragedy has occurred.

REFERENCES

Arce, A. A., Vergare, M. J. (1984). Identifying and characterizing the mentally ill among the homeless. In H. R. Lamb (Ed.), *The homeless mentally ill*. Washington, DC: American Psychiatric Association.

Barrow, S. M. (1988). *Linking mentally ill homeless clients to psychiatric treatment services: The experience of five CSS programs*. New York: New York State Psychiatric Institute.

Bassuk, E. L. (1984). The homelessness problem. *Scientific American, 251*, 40–45

Hopper, K., Hamberg, J. (1986). *The making of America's homeless: From skid row poor to new poor*. New York: Community Service Society.

Koegel P. (1992). Understanding homelessness: An ethnographic approach. In R. I. Jahiel (Ed.), *Homelessness: A prevention-oriented approach*. Baltimore: Johns Hopkins University Press.

Koegel, P., & Burnam, M. A. (1992). Issues in the assessment of mental disorders among the homeless: An empirical approach. In M. Robertson & M. Greenblatt (Eds.), *Homelessness: The national perspective*. New York: Plenum Press.

Koegel, P., Burnam, M. A., & Farr, R. K. (1988). The prevalence of specific psychiatric disorders among homeless individuals in the inner-city of Los Angeles. *Archives of General Psychiatry, 45*, 1085–1092

Lamb, H. R. (1984). Deinstitutionalization and the homeless mentally ill. In H. R. Lamb (Ed.), *The homeless mentally ill*. Washington, DC: American Psychiatric Association.

Morrissey, J. P., & Dennis, D. (1986). *NIMH-funded research concerning homeless mentally ill persons: Implications for policy and practice*. Rockville, MD: National Institute of Mental Health.

Robertson, M. J. (in press). Mental disorder, homelessness, and barriers to services: A review of the empirical literature. In R. I. Jahiel (Ed.), *Homelessness: A prevention-oriented approach*. Baltimore: Johns Hopkins University Press.

Rog, D. J., Andranovich, G. D., & Rosenblum, S. (1987). *Intensive case management for persons who are homeless and mentally ill*. Washington, DC: Cosmos Corporation.

Segal, S., Baumohl, J., & Johnson, E. (1977). Falling through the cracks: Mental disorder and social margin in a young vagrant population. *Social Problems, 24*, 387–400.

Tessler, R. C., & Dennis, D. L. (1989). A synthesis of NIMH-funded research concerning persons who are homeless and mentally ill. Rockville, MD: National Institute of Mental Health.

Mental Health Considerations In Homeless Families: Intake, Diagnoses, and Treatment

17

Joanne Jubelier

CHAPTER HIGHLIGHTS

- Homelessness is associated with several psychological losses; families lose their sense of identity, parents lose their sense of competency, and children lose the idea of home.
- Mental health services for homeless families seek out families where they live, are crisis oriented, and should be part of a multidiciplinary team.
- In the homeless setting, a brief intake process, based on subjective and objective observations, is used to determine a family's level of function or dysfunction.
- A developmental and psychosocial history are crucial elements in assessing the mental health of homeless children.
- Generally, evaluation of homeless families should be based on their level of function or dysfunction rather than traditional psychiatric diagnoses.
- Psychiatric diagnoses are, however, appropriate for parents in need of medications or special referral services and especially children in need of early intervention and symptom-specific treatment.
- A diagnosis of posttraumatic stress disorder might appropriately be applied to homeless children.
- Treatment for homeless parents and children should include both counseling and case management services.

INTRODUCTION

The number of homeless female single-parent families is a growing problem nationally and a cause of concern among mental health professionals. Numerous psychological problems, such as mental illness, drug abuse, and family disruptions, are prevalent among poor families (Saxe, Cross, & Silverman, 1988). These psychological problems may be even more common in homeless families (Bassuk & Rosenberg 1988; Bassuk, 1986b; Wood, 1989).

Many homeless parents have limited or no extended family or support systems (Hutchinson, Searight, & Stretch, 1986; McChesney, 1989). They come from chronically unstable and economically impoverished backgrounds, characterized by broken homes, substance abuse, family violence, or child abuse and foster placement.

Homelessness is associated with a series of psychological losses for the parent and the child. Although these are experienced differently by each family, overall, the trauma filters down from parent to child. For the parent, homelessness is a time filled with anger, frustration and humiliation. The privacy of family life, along with its unique norms and rules, has been disrupted. This becomes readily apparent when homeless families go to a shelter for transitional housing. The family loses a sense of identity, and the parent loses autonomy as well as a sense of competency and authority. All of these factors contribute to a sense of being out of control of one's own life for adult and child alike.

The disruption caused by homelessness is truly traumatizing for children because they have less cognitive ability to understand fully all that is happening and why. Furthermore, their parents are often likely to displace their anger and frustration onto them. This displacement may take the form of neglectful or increased demands on the children to behave or assume responsibilities that are unrealistic or that are an unfair burden to the child. Intense irritation and verbal abuse often occur if the child does not conform. This, in turn, can cause or exacerbate psychological symptoms in homeless children.

For homeless children, the loss of their home or apartment, neighborhood, and school contribute to the loss of the *idea* of home, of a sense of place. This, in turn, creates a loss of stability and continuity that all children need to thrive physically as well as emotionally. Homeless children are deprived of the psychological foundations needed to master their age-appropriate developmental tasks. Instead, there is risk, incomprehension, and unpredictability, all of which cause a very basic loss of self-control and self-esteem.

This all-encompassing loss of the familiar and the predictable typically includes the loss of significant others, such as the loss of a male adult, other family members, friends, and neighbors. These losses, as well as those described earlier, can impact on the family as intensely as the physical sufferings arising from homelessness.

This chapter deals with the ways in which clinicians and service agencies might intervene to stabilize and treat the mental health needs of homeless single-parent female families. General considerations will be discussed first, followed by a discussion of intake, diagnosis, and treatment.

GENERAL STABILIZATION AND TREATMENT CONSIDERATIONS

The provision of mental health services to homeless families differs from services provided non-homeless families in several respects. First, at least in the initial intervention, mental health providers must, as part of an outreach team, seek out homeless families where they live—in shelters, parks, or on the streets.

Second, these initial interventions are, by necessity, going to be crisis-oriented because any family experiencing the nightmare of homelessness is in a state of crisis requiring emergency or very directive measures (i.e., telling the family what to do) to assist in stabilization. Clinicians do not have the luxury of knowing a family or observing family dynamics over time before pursuing interventions.

Third, mental health services to homeless families are most effective as part of a broad-based effort to address the physical, medical, psychological, social, and economic sources of family instability with the aim of ameliorating and subsequently changing the family's overall situation. This includes addressing not only the family's medical and psychological needs, but also food and housing entitlements as well as child care, educational, legal, and job-related requirements. Thus, the best way to attend to the mental health needs of homeless families is by providing comprehensive care that addresses the biopsychosocial needs of the family. For many homeless families, this approach will be psychotherapeutic and may be all the mental health services they need even if no formal, ongoing counseling occurs.

Fourth, the mental health practitioner should be part of a multi-disciplinary team that includes clinicians of both physical and mental health, as well as a case manager or family advocate. This multi-disciplinary approach can provide needed support and insight for the clinician and a multiperspective view of diagnosis and treatment planning for each family. Whenever possible, to maintain continuity of care, the family should be assigned one counselor from initial contact to termination of whatever treatment ensues.

Fifth, mental health interventions with this population always involve case management.[1] In settings where a case manager or family advocate is unavailable, the mental health counselor should assume these responsibilities, thereby expanding the traditional psychotherapeutic role. In settings where such services can be provided by others, the counselor should communicate often with the case manager to facilitate family stabilization.

Finally, homeless families often need assistance in obtaining follow-up care after the initial intervention. At a minimum, maps and bus tokens for transportation can facilitate follow-through on appointments. Clinicians should, whenever possible, make referral connections for, and transition the family into, the referral agency by calling and making the first appointment, or giving the client a specific person to talk to at each agency. These measures can greatly increase compliance.

FAMILY INTAKE

The intake process can be one of the most significant mental health interventions. It should consist of important data gathering both on the family as a whole and each family member separately. The intake process should also initiate a program of crisis intervention and case management that stabilizes the family and provides it with new tools for survival.

---

[1]Case management means interventions that increase "access to those human services needed to resolve immediate and longer-term needs" (See chapter 3 by Cousineau, Casanova, and Erlenbusch on case management). Case management should go beyond the simple provision of information and referral; it is an active process involving the provider as the family's best and most immediate advocate. This is not only psychotherapeutic itself but also the best kind of assistance that can be provided to homeless families.

The initial intake must provide for privacy. Because the conditions under which homeless families are seen can be noisy and crowded (especially in a shelter), setting up partitions is an essential minimum. If possible, intakes should be performed in private rooms large enough to accommodate an entire family, with floor space for children to play.

Generally, given the conditions under which homeless families are seen clinically—in a shelter or on the streets—a rather speedy and modified intake that addresses the family's most immediate and important concerns is likely to occur. For those clinicians who are able to do a more traditional intake, Table 17.1 summarizes the relevant areas to be covered. Although unlikely, a detailed intake could be truly beneficial because the crisis of homelessness might present the family with the first opportunity for comprehensive evaluation and treatment. An edited copy of the assessment should be made available to parents so that, even if they leave the area, they can follow through on the recommendations at a later date.

Table 17.1 Intake of Homeless Families

Purpose:
Comprehensive collection of data
Initiation of relevant crisis or case management interventions
Generate relevant diagnoses and treatment plan
Focus:
Short-term: Propose and implement immediate treatment plan to address acute problems (obtaining shelter, applying for welfare assistance or Supplemental Security Income, and getting medical attention)
Long-term: Obtain detailed family history to identify and treat ongoing or chronic problems (identifying and treating substance abuse, parent-child problems, depression, developmental delays, etc.)
Data collection:
Mother: Identifying data, reasons for homelessness, and other presenting problems
    Pyschosocial history
    Medical history
    Summary (include both objective and subjective data)
Child: Identifying data, presenting problems
    Developmental history
    Psychosocial history
    Medical history
    Summary (include both objective and subjective data)

A brief intake should include a synthesis of objective data (see Table 17.1) with the clinician's subjective observations or impressions. This latter material can be especially relevant by giving the therapist diagnostic insight into each family member, into the family's problems as a whole, and into its level of dysfunction.

Thus, the intake should be used as a process to determine ultimately a family's level of function or dysfunction. A brief model for parent and child evaluations will now be discussed.

FAMILY INTAKE: PARENTS

The clinician should assess how the family presents physically and psychologically. This assessment should include the parent's appearance, level of cleanliness, and tidiness;[2] affective state and mental status;[3] capacity to relate to the children and to the clinician; and level of insight and ability to conceptualize problems and generate solutions.

At a minimum, the clinician should explore the following areas of the mother's psychosocial history: family of origin (with special emphasis placed on family stability, both economically and interpersonally), educational level, employment history, and—most important—relationships with significant others (especially the biological fathers[s] of her children and her relationship with her own parents). If not mentioned, the therapist should query the mother on any history of child abuse (physical or sexual), or any separations from her family as a child and reasons for them (for example, foster placement owing to abuse). Information regarding a history of substance abuse and of family violence (past or present) should also be gathered.

Although some families are homeless because of economic marginality or impoverishment caused by a death, chronic illness, or a job loss, many others are homeless because they have a multigenerational history of psychosocial instability, compounding the problems of poverty.

When long-term psychological problems occur, homelessness is best addressed by not only helping the family find housing and

---

[2]It is surprising that even in a shelter environment, hygiene can be very revealing of the level of family function or dysfunction. The more psychologically disturbed the mother, the less able she is to keep herself and her children neat and clean.

[3]A formal examination is not recommended unless in the rare instance psychosis is suspected as a diagnosis.

obtain entitlements, but also by providing case management and psychological counseling to the fullest degree possible (Bassuk, 1986a). (See Table 17.2 for a list of specific interventions.)

Intake Summary

The material should be organized as a series of mental health formulations or hyptheses generating psychological explanations for those problems, acute and chronic, relevant to the current situation. The material should include the clinician's understanding of what has gone on previously in the parent's life, her current problems, as well as what might be expected in the future.

Table 17.2 Range of Services for Homeless Parents and Children

	Counseling services	Case management services
Parents:	Family therapy	Ongoing drug program
	Individual therapy	(12-step program)
	Multifamily group therapy	Drop-in education classes
	Parent's support group	Parent educational group
	Parent-child abuse-neglect group	Job advocacy, counseling
	Parent-child group	Money management classes
	Women's group	Continuing education
	Detoxification program	Family planning
Children:	Family therapy	Legal aid
	Individual therapy	Day care or after-school care
	Group therapy	Big Brothers, Big Sisters, Scouts
	Art therapy	Drug prevention, counseling
	Play therapy	Educational therapy
	Infant stimulation	Educational advocacy
		Special class placements
		Speech and language therapy
		Psychodiagnostic testing and treatment for learning disabilities, attention deficit disorders, developmental disorders

The following variables should be considered in synthesizing the material into a relevant dynamic formulation:

- Identifying the mother's individual psychopathology (i.e., arriving at a psychiatric diagnosis if relevant to both understanding and assisting the parent in a positive direction)
- Assessing the environmental factors that cause or exacerbate the parent's problems (e.g., abandonment by husband, recent move to a new city, loss of a job, no support system or extended family)
- Assessing the risk factors that can complicate the current picture (e.g. drug problems, family violence, history of arrests, chronic unemployment, chronic welfare assistance, etc.)

FAMILY INTAKE: CHILDREN

The level of cleanliness and tidiness can again be helpful indexes of the family's, especially the parent's, ability to function positively despite major ongoing stress. Physical appearance can also be an important indicator of whether neglect is occurring.

Observations regarding family relationships also provide important clues to the family's level of functioning and the degree to which some of its problems might be chronic. In this regard, the following are important: how the child(ren) relates to the mother, how she relates to each child, how they relate to each other, and how each relates to the clinician.[4]

Finally, the clinician should assess each child's affective state, especially to identify children suffering from acute anxiety, anger, or depression. Behavioral indexes are also important indicators of underlying psychological conditions in children. Observations of regressive behaviors, for example, can indicate that a child is either frankly developmentally delayed or suffering from acute anxiety causing temporary loss of certain developemental gains (e.g., speech or toilet training).[5] Additionally, the child's verbal abilities may be a good

---

[4]For example, is one child the family caretaker (i.e., the pseudomature child)? Is one scapegoated or treated with hostility? Do the children constantly bicker or fight aggressively with each other? Regarding interactions with the clinician, do any want constant attention or affection? Are any inaccessible emotionally?

[5]Other behavioral manifestations of underlying psychological conditions are constant activity and fidgeting, which may indicate anxiety or hyperactivity; oppositionalism, which may indicate anger or depression; and passivity, which may be an indicator of depression, anxiety, or anger.

index of his or her cognitive abilities, and his or her ability to understand what is happening and why.

Because homelessness can disrupt or hinder a child's physical or psychological development, whenever possible, clinicians should take both a developmental and psychosocial history in addition to obtaining medical information.[6]

Developmental History

The interviewing circumstances will probably mitigate against obtaining a full developmental history. If possible, however, a detailed developmental history is recommended as many homeless children are developmentally delayed in one or a combination of areas (Bassuk & Rubin, 1987; Bassuk, Rubin, & Lauriat, 1986; Wood, 1989b). The history should cover the child's attainment of crawling, walking, talking, toilet training; information on motor abilities (both gross and fine motor); cognitive abilities (i.e., the ability to understand his or her experience and to verbally express it); and school performance. Depending on the age of the child, clinicians may want to consider administering the brief form of the DDST (Frankenburg, Goldstein, & Camp, 1971) as part of the intake process as well as the Bender-Gestalt Developmental Test for Young Children (Koppitz, 1963, 1975) and the Kinetic Family Drawing (Burns, 1987), but only if there is enough training and supervision to warrant proper administration and interpretation.[7] (See Bassuk & Rubin, 1987, for information on other tests.)

---

[6]If a current medical record exists, the clinician should request a copy for the chart. Otherwise, a brief history of all medical problems should be taken including information on medications and hospitalizations.

[7]On suspected developmental delays, use of the DDST in its abbreviated form can be helpful because its administration is brief (5–10 minutes) and relies more on clinical observations than on parental report. If indicated, the clinician should refer the child for a complete diagnostic evaluation including neuropsychological testing if relevant.

The Bender-Gestalt test can be useful in identifying the presence of visual-perceptual problems as well as difficulties in cognitive and emotional organizational skills.

The Kinetic Family Drawing is a projective tool allowing the clinician entry into the child's psychological world. The resulting information is a condensation of experiences with the self, the family, and other important people, and the world at large. It is simple to administer and requires only paper and crayons or pencil.

Psychosocial History

This part of the assessment should focus on the child's emotional development, on his or her experience growing up within the family, and on his or her relationships with significant others outside of the family (e.g., at day care, any school setting, foster care, etc.). The clinician should ask about any previous separations and the reasons for them. Special attention should be paid to a history, before homelessness, of ongoing emotional and behavioral problems such as excessive withdrawn behavior, crying or shyness, oppositionalism, aggressiveness, or repeated ongoing temper tantrums. These symptoms point to the possibility of chronic, unresolved problems within the family as well as ongoing disturbance within the child.

Intake Summary

Clinical data relevant to the clinician's understanding of the child's psychological experience should be condensed and synthesized with the following guidelines in mind:

- Identification of the child's individual psychopathology, if relevant
- Assessment of identifiable environmental factors that can cause or increase the child's psychological problems (ongoing poverty, chronic medical problems, early separations)
- Assessment of relevant risk factors and their impact on the child's level of functioning (e.g., parental substance abuse; child abuse, endangerment, or neglect; family disorganization; and other impediments to diminishing the crisis of homelessness)

DIAGNOSTIC CONSIDERATIONS

The final components of the assessment process should generate tentative or working diagnoses and treatment recommendations. This is the most difficult part of the process because it requires the clinician to synthesize data relevant to each family member's history into a cohesive clinical picture of the family. Each homeless family can be evaluated in two ways: (a) by its level of function or dysfunction; or (b) by use of traditional diagnoses from the *Diagnostic and Statistical Manual of Mental Disorders* (DSM III-R) (American Psychiatric Association, 1987) when relevant and appropriate.

Generally speaking, because of the transient nature of this population and limited time, space, and staff, clinicians might consider evaluating a family by its level of function or dysfunction. If there is significant dysfunction, either within a family member or the family at large, the clinician might extend the evaluation period to do a more complete diagnostic work-up.

Use of traditional psychiatric diagnoses to describe homeless family members may not be helpful. Before using traditional diagnoses for homeless families, clinicians should ask the following questions:

- To what use will the diagnosis be put?
- Will its use aid not only in understanding but also in intervention?
- Is its use reliable or valid given the impact of homelessness (on the individual or the family) as both an unusual circumstance and an ongoing stressor? If so, which diagnoses might be applicable?
- Would the same diagnosis pertain months after homelessness is resolved?

The use of traditional diagnoses may be more relevant in the case of homeless children than their parents, as discussed subsequently.

Traditional Diagnoses: Parents

Basically, differential diagnoses will be most important and effective for parents when medication, hospitalization, day treatment, or detoxification are considerations. Thus, care should be given to identifying substance abuse, thought disorders, mood disorders, and paranoid states. Anxiety disorders and/or personality disorders are likely to occur with frequency, but knowing the exact personality disorder probably will not assist the treatment strategy or final outcome. When homeless women are undergoing such profound distress, it seems inappropriate to attach psychiatric labels unless it is clear that the external stressors are exacerbating an underlying condition as opposed to impeding one's true ability to function in the world.[8]

---

[8]For example, posttraumatic stress disorder also may be common in this population. Caution is required in making differential diagnoses. Correlative disorders, such as depression, sleep disturbances, brief reactive psychoses, or somatiform disorders can coexist. In case of posttraumatic stress disorder, some psychological symptoms, which initially suggest a more serious disorder, may actually reflect severe anxiety resulting from transient, situational stressors of an acute nature. Posttraumatic stress disorder also needs to be differentiated from the common crisis reaction.

Traditional Diagnoses: Children

The use of psychiatric diagnoses with respect to children, conversely, can be especially useful if it can generate early identification and symptom-specific treatment. If the crisis of homelessness provides an opportunity to give troubled children the help they sorely need, then traditional diagnostic categorization is a useful vehicle to effect the process. The most relevant diagnoses are those that describe the common disorders observed in homeless children: anxiety disorders and posttraumatic stress disorder, dysthymia (depression), disruptive behavior disorder, elimination and developmental disorders, and, possibly, elective mutism. A series of different types of treatment, both in theoretical orientation (e.g., psychodynamic, behavioral) and modality (e.g., individual, group) can be appropriate given the needs of each child. Thus, there is not necessarily one correct treatment of choice for any disorder mentioned earlier.[9] A correct diagnosis is essential for proper treatment, however.

Homelessness itself, in addition to whatever psychological problems existed in the family previously, is most likely a major causative factor in several prevalent and overlapping conditions found in these children, especially the anxiety disorders and posttraumatic stress disorder. It is common to find the younger homeless child suffering from separation anxiety disorder especially regarding the following criteria, listed in the DSM-III-R (American Psychiatric Association, 1987, p. 61):

- Unrealistic and persistent worry about possible harm befalling major attachment figures, or fear that they will leave and not return
- Persistent reluctance or refusal to go to sleep without being near a major attachment figure or to go to sleep away from home
- Persistent avoidance of being alone including "clinging" to and "shadowing" major attachment figures
- repeated nightmares involving the theme of separation
- recurrent signs or complaints of excessive distress in anticipation of separation from major attachment figures (e.g., temper tantrums or crying, pleading with parents not to leave)

---

[9]The use of medications poses a different set of considerations and will not be discussed here.

For the child who is 2 1/2 years or older, anxiety may additionally manifest itself through an avoidant disorder, that is "excessive shrinking from contact with unfamiliar people, for a period of six months or longer, sufficiently severe to interfere with social functioning in peer relationships" (American Psychiatric Association, 1987, p. 62).

Although there appears to be no research data in the area, the diagnosis of posttraumatic stress disorder might appropriately be used for many of the children suffering from the trauma of homelessness.[10] The condition is described in the DSM-III-R as one in which the person experiences an event that is "outside the range of usual human experience and that would be markedly distressing to almost anyone e.g., as sudden destruction of one's home or community" (American Psychiatric Association, 1987, p. 250). The following are some of the common criteria from the DSM-III-R that suggest this syndrome in homeless children:

- Markedly diminished interest in significant activities (in young children, loss of recently acquired developmental skills such as toilet training or language skills)
- Feeling of detachment or estrangement from others
- Restricted range of affect (e.g., unable to have loving feelings)
- Difficulty falling or staying asleep
- Irritability or outbursts of anger
- Difficulty concentrating
- Hypervigilance
- Exaggerated startle response

As this list of symptoms illustrates, the trauma of homelessness makes differential diagnosis quite complicated. This is particularly true when it comes to differentiating posttraumatic stress disorder from other diagnoses of anxiety disorders, the disruptive behavior disorders, and the developmental disorders.

Additionally, the clinician should also expect to see many problems associated with the developmental disorders (i.e., mental retardation, academic skills, language and speech, or motor skills). Many homeless children have had little stimulation within the family to promote the development of cognitive and language skills. In

---

[10]For more specifics on how to make this diagnosis correctly, please see DSM-III-R (American Psychiatric Association, 1987, pp. 247–251).

addition, they lack input from school, where attendance is usually discontinuous at best.

In summary, given the prospects of early intervention, the use of DSM III-R diagnoses is often appropriate for homeless children. Given the fluidity and emotional complexity of childhood development, and given the presence of severe environmental stressors, however, the task of making discrete diagnoses is extremely difficult. The difficulty is compounded by two issues: one or a combination of diagnostic conditions might be applicable to one individual; and the diagnoses must be considered in interaction with family dynamics (and possible dysfunction) as well as with other current risk or environmental stressors the child is encountering.[11]

Any of the diagnostic problems mentioned earlier can cause or perpetuate family dysfunction through impaired parent-child and sibling relationships. Each of these problems can impact negatively on the entire family's ability to function as a unit. Additionally, behavioral manifestations of his or her problems can predispose the homeless child to be at risk for abuse or neglect. Thus, unless there is some need to make an immediate psychiatric diagnosis, the initial contact time should be used to assess each homeless family for its capacity to function as a cohesive unit rather than to make a psychiatric diagnosis.

TREATMENT CONSIDERATIONS

Generally, child and family psychotherapy issues tend to be the same across socioeconomic lines. All families, at one time or another experience parent-child problems such as problems in parental limit setting and discipline, separation anxiety in the young child, or rebellion in the teenager. What differs for homeless families is the initial treatment approach, one that will always require crisis intervention, case management, and outreach into the community.

In traditional family therapy, middle- and upper-middle class families come to a clinic or clinician's office for psychotherapy. This is also true of the working poor who have permanent shelter, although other considerations such as clinic hours, child care, and

---

[11]For more information on the interaction between a child's mental health, low socioeconomic status, and environmental risk factors, see Tuma (1989).

transportation become important concerns. In working with homeless families, the clinic and clinician often go to the family where they live, in a park, or, it is hoped, some form of transitional shelter. The ultimate goal is to bring the family to the clinic and to assist the family in complying with recommendations so it can get the full assistance it deserves. The specific treatment approaches, however, will vary according to the needs and problems within any given family as well as to its level of function or dysfunction. The range of specific family and child services that might be used are listed in Table 17.2.

As can be seen from the parent-child counseling and case management services listed in Table 17.2, separate approaches are required for parents and children. In general, however, a basic dual-intervention approach is recommended for all homeless families that are stablized enough to participate in treatment on a regular basis— family therapy accompanied by individual counseling for the mother.

Family therapy contains within it the opportunity to provide a wide array of interventions aimed at addressing both individual and family psychopathology as well as parent education and modeling by the clinician to improve communication skills, empathy, limit setting, and discipline. Successful interventions into the family system generally lead to feelings of relief and support. This is especially necessary for homeless parents, who are burdened with innumerable responsibilities in addition to attending to the emotional life of the family.

Because emotional support is otherwise limited or nonexistent for homeless mothers, individual counseling can contribute greatly to the parent's self-esteem while addressing the many chronic sources of deprivation and instability contributing to her family's dysfunction.

Despite many limitations (e.g., limited staff, time, and money to provide services to the families), effective and helpful interventions can still be made (Bassuk, 1986b). The most important initial treatment is usually conducted by the outreach team. These community interventions necessitate ongoing liaison between the on-site team, the team's agency, and other service providers.

Charting can be a problem on site, and each service provider should organize a system to ensure continuity of care. Whatever procedure is used, notations, which are signed and dated, must be made consistently. Notations include information on who was seen, what was discussed (in a brief and general way to protect confidentiality), and any recommendations made to the family. The latter should be as specific as possible so that the case manager or other agency personnel can assist in follow-through.

Optimally, family therapy should be integrated with crisis intervention and case management at the outset, especially with the more dysfunctional families. Given the transient nature of homelessness and family disorganization, however, psychotherapy on an ongoing basis is unlikely to occur until a stable dwelling has been found. Unfortunately, the opportunity to use psychotherapy as a change agent (by helping families to follow through with treatment recommendations so that new understandings and methods of dealing with old problems can develop) is least likely to occur when it is needed the most.

A discussion of treatment considerations cannot be complete without addressing two barriers to the provision of treatment to homeless families. First is the limited availability of actual services that can be provided either free of charge or at reduced fee. A scarcity of mental health services for children exists nationwide (Inouye, 1988; Saxe et al., 1988; Tuma, 1989). The scarcity is particularly acute for homeless families.

The second problem is patient compliance. Homeless families most in need of family treatment and case management (i.e., the multigenerational dysfunctional family) are least likely to obtain available services because of poor compliance. These homeless families need volunteers who can function both as adoptive parents and family advocates, unless a case manager is actively involved. Such volunteers will, by their attention and assistance (e.g., in child care, transportation, accompanying members through contacts with large institutions, making calls, etc.), provide and facilitate treatment.[12]

CONCLUSION

The nightmare of family homelessness may be the first opportunity for comprehensive biopsychosocial interventions (psychological, economic, educational, vocational, social, and medical), especially

---

[12]Volunteers can be recruited from various civic and religious organizations. Needless to say, a volunteer of this sort could also be of tremendous support to the responsible clinician, sharing in many of the case management aspects and thereby freeing the clinician's time and reducing stress.

for the multigenerational dysfunctional family. These interventions will initially entail outreach by a multidisciplinary team of clinicians.

Comprehensive interventions will also entail an expanded and flexible approach to one's role as a practitioner. For the mental health clinician, counseling, by necessity, will include a case management orientation (even if a case manager participates) so that family change can occur in all areas where assistance is needed. Moreover, whatever one's psychotherapeutic orientation, helping the family to address and satisfy basic needs will be instrumental in helping the family to stabilize psychologically.

The assessment process (i.e., intake, diagnosis, and treatment recommendations) will most likely be brief, and the clinician should make whatever interventions are needed to lessen the current crisis. Unless psychiatric diagnoses are warranted, as is sometimes the case in treating homeless children, the clinician's time will be better spent assessing the family's general level of function or dysfunction, and directing interventions toward empowering the family and building esteem.

Many homeless children are severely troubled emotionally, either as a consequence of homelessness, or as a result of chronic family dysfunction and poverty. These children may also be disabled developmentally, and may have never attended public school or have done so sporadically. Thus, early identification and treatment of the many psychosocial problems of homeless children are crucial. Unfortunately, whatever psychiatric diagnoses pertain, it is highly probable that homeless children, once stabilized, will continue to suffer from the physical and emotional trauma caused by homelessness.

The potential implications of so many physically and psychologically damaged homeless children are staggering: family homelessness will take its toll on our future labor force, welfare, foster care, and criminal justice systems. Additionally, we are likely to have a large population of multidisabled "have nots," many of whom were homeless from birth, contributing to an ever-increasing breach between advantaged and disadvantaged Americans.

Service-enriched low-income housing, providing a broad array of community-based social, medical, and psychological support, is needed to stop the vicious cycle of homelessness. Only by investing in today's homeless population can we prevent the tragedy of a new generation of dysfunctional homeless families.

REFERENCES

American Psychiatric Association. (1987). *Diagnostic and statistical manual of mental disorders* (3rd ed., rev.). Washington DC: Author.

Bassuk, E. L. (1986a, Fall). Homeless families: Assessing a new American tragedy. *Generics, 48–57.*

Bassuk, E. L. (1986b). "Homeless families: Single mothers and their children in Boston shelters. In *The Mental Health Needs of Homeless Persons: New Directions for Mental Health Services* (pp. 45–53).

Bassuk, E. L., & Rubin, L. (1987). Homeless children: A neglected population. *American Journal of Orthopsychiatry, 57,* 279–286.

Bassuk, E. L., Rubin, L., & Lauriat, A. (1986). Characteristics of sheltered homeless families. *American Journal of Public Health, 76,* 1097–1101

Bassuk, E. L., & Rosenberg, L. (1988). Why does family homelessness occur? A case-control study. *American Journal of Public Health, 78,* 783–788.

Burns, R. C. (1987). Self-growth in families: Kinetic family drawings (K-F-D). In *Research and application.* Brunner Mazel.

Frankenburg, W. K., Goldstein, A., & Camp, B. (1971). The revised Denver developmental screening test: Its accuracy as a screening instrument. *Journal of Pediatrics, 79,* 988–995.

Hutchinson, W. J., Searight, P., & Stretch, J. J. (1986, November-December). Multidimentional networking: A response to the needs of homeless families. *Social Work,* 427–430.

Inouye, D. (1988). Children's mental health issues. *American Psychologist, 43,* 813–16.

Koppitz, E. M. (1963). *Bender Gestalt test for young children:* New York: Grune & Stratton.

Koppitz, E. M. (1975). *Bender Gestalt test for young children, Vol. 2. Research and applications, 1963–1973.* New York: Grune & Stratton.

McChesney, K. Y. (1989, August). *Absence of a safety net for homeless families.* Paper presented at the annual meeting of American Sociological Association, San Francisco.

Saxe, L., Cross, T., & Silverman, N. (1988). Children's mental health: The gap between what we know and what we do. *American Psychologist, 43,* 800–807.

Tuma, J. M. (1989). Mental health services for children: The state-of-the-art. *American Psychologist, 44,* 188–196.

Wood, D. (1989). Homeless children: Their evaluation and treatment. *Journal of Pediatric Health Care, 3,* 194–199.

Index

"The Ability to Pay Plan" (ATP), 33
Abscess, in homeless, 146–147
Acquired immunodeficiency syndrome (AIDS), 6, 32, 36, 56, 58, 63, 67, 72, 93, 151
Acute health problems, in homeless, 55–56
Advocacy
  by case managers, 33
  definition, 58
  in HIV infection, 118
  by outreach health care services, 58
AIDS. *See* Acquired immunodeficiency syndrome, *and* Human immunodeficiency virus (HIV) in homeless
AIDS-related complex (ARC), 117, 120
Aid to Families with Dependent Children (AFDC), 32
Alcohol abuse, 97–101
  assessment, 97
  educating shelter staff about, 59
  history and clinical manifestations, 98–99
  hypothermia and, 162
  incidence of, 93
  laboratory abnormalities associated with ingestion of ethanol, 100t
  laboratory assessment, 99–100
  mentally ill and, 239
  pathological conditions associated with chronic ethanol consumption, 98t
  treatment, 100–101
American Academy of Pediatrics, 203, 208

AZT, 117, 123, 129–130

Birth control, for homeless, 191
Bites, in homeless, 148
Body lice, in homeless, 153–154
  treatment for, 154–155
Boston Health Care for the Homeless Program, 115
Breast examinations, 67–68
Burns, 149

Cancer screening, 67–68
Case management
  barriers to, 32–35
  functions of, 36–45
  for homeless families, 30–45
  populations served by, 32
Case manager(s)
  as advocate, 33
  attitudes and biases of, 34
  burnout of, 44
  case review by, 42
  in crisis intervention, 37–40
  distrust of, by homeless, 34–35
  follow-up by, 43
  health care model and, 35–36
  making effective referrals, 41–42
  networking by, 44
  role of, 31
  social change and, 43
  as term, 31
Case review, 42
Cellulitis, 146
Child abuse
  educating shelter staff about, 58–59
  preventing, 57
  screening for, 205–206

273

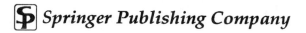 *Springer Publishing Company*

HEALTH CARE OF HOMELESS PEOPLE

Philip W. Brickner, MD, **Linda K. Scharer**, MUP, **Barbara Conanan**, RN, MS, **Alexander Elvy**, MSW, and **Marianne Savarese**, RN, BSN, *all of St. Vincent's Hospital, New York*, Editors

"It is a major contribution to the understanding of homelessness and its impact on delivery of health care services and should be required reading in every school of social work in the country as well as in medical, nursing, and health care administration curricula." —**Social Work in Health Care**

Partial Contents: Health Issues in the Care of the Homeless, *P.W. Brickner*. Infestations: Scabies and Lice, *R.W. Green*. Exposure: Thermoregulatory Disorders in the Homeless Patient, *L. Goldfrank*. Trauma: With the Example of San Francisco's Shelter Programs, *J.T. Kelly*. Alcoholism and the Homeless, *R. Morgan et al*. Psychiatry and Homelessness: Problems and Programs, *S.L. Kellermann et al*. The Toll of Deinstitutionalization, *K. Flynn*. Access to Care, *A. Elvy*. Health Care Teams in Work with the Homeless, *M. Savarese*. Working with Hospitals, *L.K. Scharer and B. Price*. Health Care and the Homeless: Access to Benefits, *S. Crystal*. Washington, D.C.: The Zacchaeus Clinic—A Model of Health Care for Homeless Persons, *E. Bargmann*.

A United Hospital Fund Book
1985   349pp   0-8261-4990-1   hardcover

COMMUNITY HEALTH NURSING
Theory and Practice

Carl O. Helvie, RN, DrPH, *Old Dominion University, Norfolk, Virginia*

This important volume meets the critical need for a single sourcebook incorporating theory, process, and clinical practice tools. Dr. Helvie has crafted a book that serves both undergraduate and graduate-level nursing students, in addition to staff nurses new to community health nursing.

Partial Contents: Introduction to Community Health Nursing Theory. Community Health Nursing Theory and the Family. Relating and Communicating with Clients. Concepts in Health and Epidemiology. Understanding Crisis and Disaster: Useful Concepts and Theories. Clinical Practice Tools—Assessment; Planning; Selected Community Health Nursing Interventions; Evaluation Tools; Useful Resources.

1991   476pp   0-8261-6550-8   hardcover